MW01285255

"This book is brilliant, I love it. It so obviously reflects a deep understanding of the barriers people face and compassionate ways to overcome them. Every chapter offers strategies that can help you today, with the body you have and the challenges you face. Every page has an insight that can help you find joy in movement (or get you moving). It's the most insightful guide to getting moving I've ever read."—**Kelly McGonigal**, author of *The Joy of Movement*

"This book is the nudge you need and will get you rethinking your relationship to movement entirely. You'll want to keep this one on your shelf to reference again and again."—**Manoush Zomorodi**, host of NPR's *TED Radio Hour* and *Body Electric*

"[A] remarkable and timely book that applies the powerful tools of modern psychological science to help readers overcome the mental and emotional barriers to movement, [by] connecting actions to deeply held values rather than temporary motivations or fearful but often incorrect predictions.

What stands out most to me is the book's innovative choice to highlight and undermine excessive reason-giving: a topic I've long found fascinating and the original basis of my own research on ACT and psychological flexibility four decades ago. It's wonderful to see reason-giving addressed in such a powerful, compassionate, and effective way. I can think of no book ever, in any area, that has explored it so thoroughly and artfully.

As you read it you will discover that this book is not really just for those who want to exercise. It's for anyone seeking a richer, more intentional relationship with their mind, body, and values. Whether you're a fitness professional, mental health practitioner, or someone who just wants to get unstuck, this book will make a difference."—**Steven C. Hayes**, Ph.D., originator of Acceptance and Commitment Therapy; author of *Get Out of Your Mind and Into Your Life* and *A Liberated Mind*

"As a barefoot trail runner, dedicated yogi, and longtime admirer of Katy Bowman's Nutritious Movement approach, I've seen the power of physical activity. As a co-founder of Acceptance and Commitment Therapy (ACT), I also understand the psychological roadblocks to healthy movement. *I Know I Should Exercise But...*masterfully combines Diana Hill's ACT expertise with Katy Bowman's biomechanics insights. This book tackles both the physical and psychological barriers to movement, offering practical, compassionate steps to get started."—**Kelly G. Wilson**, Ph.D., Professor Emeritus, University of Mississippi, author of *Mindfulness for Two*, *Things Might Go Terribly, Horribly Wrong*, and *The Wisdom to Know the Difference*

"At long last, a book that compassionately addresses the real and often debilitating reasons that so many of us resist physical movement. From low self-esteem to high anxiety, from lack of space to obligation overload, Katy Bowman and Diana Hill leave no obstacle unturned as they clear the way for anyone and everyone who has ever wanted to get moving, but found themselves flummoxed—whether by resistance, uncertainty, distraction, or dread. A great guide for anyone longing to live in a healthier body-mind, and a fine professional toolkit for coaches, trainers, and psychologists who want to help others accomplish that goal with greater ease."—**Pilar Gerasimo**, author of *The Healthy Deviant* and Founder of Healthy Deviant U.

"[A] refreshing and empowering resource for anyone struggling to move more. Katy Bowman and Diana Hill skillfully transform guilt and resistance into joy and sustainable habits, making this a must-read for individuals and health professionals alike."—**Leigh A. Frame**, Ph.D., MHS, Chief Wellness Officer, George Washington University School of Medicine and Health Sciences

"This book has a perfect answer for every preconceived notion or excuse that may arise when it comes to exercising. It should be required reading for many of the pregnant and postpartum patients I work with, who struggle to find the time, are tired or unmotivated, or have children or partners who don't support their movement habit."—**Anietie Ukpe-Wallace**, PT, DPT, orthopedic and pelvic health physical therapist and author of *Tending to Your Womb* (Uphill Books, June 2025)

"[E]xceptionally authoritative and compassionate, *I Know I Should Exercise But…* is [also] accessible, loaded with practical tips, and just plain old fun to read! I also greatly appreciate that it's been written so that you can jump to sections that are more relevant to your own struggles or as they become more relevant to your journey.

As a research psychologist who conducts studies on physical activity, I can honestly say I found myself repeatedly highlighting sections because they were presented in either a particularly engaging, unique, or entertaining way, and I will most certainly be recommending this book to anyone who wants to exercise more but can't quite get momentum going."—**Jason Lillis**, Ph.D., Associate Professor, Warren Alpert Medical School of Brown University and co-author of *Acceptance and Commitment Therapy* and *The Diet Trap*

I Know
I **Should**
Exercise
But...

44 Reasons We Don't Move
& How to Get Over Them

By Diana Hill, Ph.D.
and Katy Bowman, M.S.

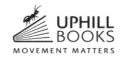

UPHILL
BOOKS
MOVEMENT MATTERS

Printed in the United States of America

First Edition, First Printing, 2025
ISBN-13: 9781943370313
Library of Congress Control Number: 2024945348
Uphill Books: uphill-books.com, Sequim, WA

Editor: Penelope Jackson
Science Editor: Andrea Graves
Text & Cover Design by: Agnes Koller, figdesign.ca
Proofreader: Kate Kennedy
Indexer: Michael Curran
Author photos by Esteban Leyva Photography (Diana) and Mahina Hawley (Katy)

The information in this book should not be used for diagnosis or treatment, or as a substitute for professional medical care. Please consult with your health care provider prior to attempting any treatment on yourself or another individual.

Publisher's Cataloging-in-Publication
(Provided by Cassidy Cataloguing Services, Inc.)

Names:	Hill, Diana, (Psychotherapy), author.	Bowman, Katy, author.
Title:	I know I should exercise, but … : 44 reasons we don't move & how to get over them / by Diana Hill, Ph.D. and Katy Bowman, M.S.
Description:	First edition.	Sequim, WA : Uphill Books, [2025]	Includes bibliographical references and index.
Identifiers	ISBN: 9781943370313 (paperback)	9781943370320 (ebook)	LCCN: 2024945348
Subjects:	LCSH: Exercise--Psychological aspects.	Physical fitness--Psychological aspects.	Self-care, Health--Psychological aspects.	Motivation (Psychology)	Body image.	Time management.	Acceptance and commitment therapy.	Movement education.	LCGFT: Self-help publications.	BISAC: HEALTH & FITNESS / Exercise / General.	PSYCHOLOGY / Psychotherapy / Cognitive Behavioral Therapy (CBT)	SELF-HELP / Self-Management / General.
Classification:	LCC: RA781 .H55 2025	DDC: 613.71--dc23

ALSO BY DIANA HILL

Wise Effort (coming in 2025)
The Self-Compassion Daily Journal
ACT Daily Journal

ALSO BY KATY BOWMAN

My Perfect Movement Plan
Rethink Your Position
Grow Wild
Dynamic Aging
Simple Steps to Foot Pain Relief
Movement Matters
Diastasis Recti
Don't Just Sit There
Whole Body Barefoot
Move Your DNA
Alignment Matters

*For everyone who has ever struggled
with moving their body in a way
that felt joyful and free*

Table of Contents

Why Can't I Make Myself Park Farther Away from the Store?

Everywhere you look there's exercise advice, but many of us struggle to follow it. Pretty much every "Easy Ways to Move More" article tells us to "just park farther away from the store," but this simple action can be hard to take, right? If parking farther away is so easy, then why do we still circle the lot to find the closest spot—sometimes for even longer than it would have taken to walk all the way across it? Did we misunderstand the assignment? Are we just lazy? Too busy? Or is something else going on?

There are actually many reasons you might not be choosing that farther parking spot. You might be prone to negative thoughts kicking in every time you try to take action (*What's the point? I'll never really change*). Maybe you're not sure how to handle the physical discomfort. You might not value getting your steps in a gross parking lot. Maybe you were simply distracted and forgot you wanted to park farther away! In all of these cases, it's not laziness, busyness, or a lack of understanding keeping us from moving; it's more about how we relate to our experiences.

If you picked up this book, you probably care about moving your body but just can't seem to make it happen regularly. On top of that, you might also feel bad or guilty when you don't move as much as you know you "should." But it really isn't as simple as it sounds. Nourishing your body with movement takes more than just telling yourself you should exercise. There are subtle and powerful psychological and contextual barriers that block many of us from getting the physical activity we want—barriers like fatigue, not having enough time, or embarrassment. Luckily, when we approach these barriers with openness and flexibility, we can find so many paths to moving our bodies well.

I (Dr. Diana Hill) am a clinical psychologist who guides individuals and organizations to become more psychologically flexible, empowering them to take action towards their values, even when life gets hard. And I (Katy Bowman) am a biomechanist and creator of Nutritious Movement, and I've spent more than two decades showing folks all the ways movement can fit into the different domains of life (not just "exercise time"), at all our ages and stages. For this book we have joined forces to support you, dear reader, in overcoming even the trickiest movement barriers, by changing your mindset around exercise.

Parking Closer…and Psychological Flexibility

We often think about flexibility in terms of our muscles and joints—for example, we need flexible hips and backs to bend over and tie our shoes. But flexibility applies to our inner world as well. Having a flexible mindset helps us see our challenges from a broader vantage point. And if we can open up to uncomfortable emotions and sensations, we can move with them, without freezing up or becoming overwhelmed. We need to be both physically and psychologically flexible to adapt and change to new situations and habits.

Psychological flexibility is a concept that comes from Acceptance and Commitment Therapy (ACT), an approach originally developed by psychologists Steven Hayes, Kirk Strosahl, and Kelly Wilson. ACT is a therapy that has been shown to be effective for everything from mental health concerns like depression and anxiety to enhancing work performance, relationship satisfaction, and health behavior change. It works by offering you skills to accept difficult thoughts and feelings, so that you can pursue actions that align with your values. Research shows that when we are psychologically flexible, not only are we more likely to be physically active, we are also more likely to keep moving in the long run.

Psychological flexibility is our ability to stay present, connect with what matters to us, and make conscious, values-driven choices, even in the face of inner obstacles. (And if you have no idea what any of that means, don't worry—we'll get to it!) There are six core processes that help loosen up the way we relate to the world and stop us from being so rigid in our thoughts and actions, and all of them work well with a big dose of self-compassion: the practice of being kind and understanding with ourselves.

The Six Core Processes of Psychological Flexibility

 1. KNOW YOUR VALUES

Your values are the deeply held principles that guide meaningful actions and life choices. The "just park farther away" advice might not work for you if you don't connect those thirty or forty steps in the parking lot to something you value personally. When it comes to taking action, we each need to connect to our deeper "why." To help you figure out yours, grab a notebook or your phone or just a few minutes in your own head to answer these questions:

- What about moving your body really matters to you?
- When do you feel the most energized doing movement?
- How would moving your body enhance important areas of your life?
- How do you want to show up in the world with the limited time you have?

- Would you walk into the grocery store differently if you knew it was the very last time you'd be able to? If so, what would change?

In the pages ahead we'll explore how to overcome motivational barriers by going inside and asking ourselves some more exploratory questions.

 ## 2. GET FLEXIBLE WITH UNHELPFUL THOUGHTS

Our minds can be the worst motivators when it comes to movement. For example, when you're circling that parking lot, your mind might say, *I should park farther away, but I'm in a hurry* or *I'll do it next time.* Or maybe your mind criticizes you when you fail to stick to your goal of walking more. As you'll hear in the pages ahead, a lot of us battle with our thoughts—we get stuck in rules, derailed by "shoulds," and easily convinced by our own excuses. And the harder we try not to think these types of thoughts, the stronger they rebound. We can spend so much time arguing with our mind about whether or not to walk that we run out of time to do it!

To overcome your mind's barriers to movement, you will learn a strategy called *cognitive flexibility.* Instead of battling your thoughts, you will practice the following:

- stepping back from your thoughts
- getting curious about how your mind works
- choosing helpful thoughts
- breaking your mind's rules on purpose

As you'll hear in the reasons people gave for not moving, self-criticism, rules, shoulds, and excuses are really common obstacles.

 ## 3. ACCEPT DISCOMFORT

Maybe you don't want to park farther away because it's uncomfortable. Maybe it's a hot day and you don't want to sweat or carry your bags that far. Or maybe you feel a bit embarrassed or anxious that you'll stand out as different if you're the only one using the way-back part of the lot.

Moving your body is likely to involve discomfort at times, in both the body and mind. In order to overcome this barrier, you will need to learn to do these things:

- tell the difference between danger and discomfort
- increase your willingness to feel a broad range of sensations and emotions
- get comfortable with feeling uncomfortable
- practice the skill of acceptance—opening up to feelings and sensations, and making space for your full experience

4. TAKE PERSPECTIVE

There are so many ways to view and interpret every situation, but often we get stuck in just one way of seeing our circumstances, ourselves, and others. Maybe you believe that walking in a parking lot doesn't count as exercise, or "I never follow through on my plans to work out." Our rigid beliefs can even become self-fulfilling prophecies; if we think we're out of shape, we don't walk very far. And the more we believe our mind's stories, the more we look for evidence to support them. In this book, you'll hear strategies to shift your perspective on yourself as a mover, and on the idea of exercise itself. You will practice a few different techniques:

- noticing when you are caught in rigid beliefs about yourself
- taking a different perspective on yourself
- seeing exercise and movement through a more flexible lens
- finding more flexible ways to move your body
- discovering how movement can help you feel more interconnected

5. BE PRESENT

Maybe you don't park farther away because, well, you just aren't paying attention! Our minds tend to wander to pretty much everything but the present moment. We get distracted or scattered and we operate on autopilot instead of being mindful and intentional in our actions. And we get so caught in our heads we forget we have a body that needs moving. In order to park farther away, we need to be present enough to remember to do it!

A lot of the solutions to movement barriers center around the skill of becoming present. You'll practice this in a few ways:

- engaging more with the present moment
- staying attuned to your body's needs
- reorienting your attention to your movement goals
- grounding yourself in the present moment with mindfulness
- savoring the good feelings that come with moving your body

 ## 6. TAKE COMMITTED ACTION

Ultimately, if you want to nourish your body with movement, you're going to need to physically do it! That means moving your body, day after day, year after year. It's a commitment to choose to move your body, and behavioral psychology offers a lot of strategies that can help you keep that commitment. Some of these strategies are small—make sure you're wearing clothes you can walk in easily—and some are strategic, like posting a reminder (a Post-it Note works well!) on your dashboard that says *Your lower back feels better when you take short walks a few times a day!*

In order to be successful at moving more, you'll try many approaches:

- making small changes that build on each other over time
- choosing movements that fit your physical ability and context
- building social support and people who are on the same page as you

- rewarding yourself so that you stay motivated
- structuring your environment to support your movement goals

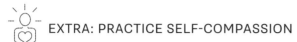 **EXTRA: PRACTICE SELF-COMPASSION**

When you're facing the task of *making* yourself park farther away, you may find that the biggest barrier is your own self-judgment. Many of us are self-critical when it comes to moving our bodies. We blame ourselves for not moving enough, for not following through. We call ourselves lazy and uncoordinated, and we point out all of our flaws. We think that being fat means we aren't healthy or can't move, or that we need to already be "in shape" to go to an exercise class. We think that shaming and strong-arming ourselves will motivate us to improve. But this approach only backfires, making us want to move less, not more!

By being self-compassionate—treating yourself with the same respect and encouragement you would someone you love—you will discover ways to move your body that are nourishing, healing, and beneficial to your whole being. **By being more self-compassionate you are more likely to move,** because you know deep down that moving is one of the kindest things you can do for yourself. With self-compassion, you will gain useful skills:

- growing a wise, encouraging inner voice
- using your compassionate inner coach to motivate you
- caring for yourself so you can better care for others
- being kind and loving towards your body

As you work through this book, you'll see examples of how to apply the six core processes of psychological flexibility as well as self-compassion to tackle your biggest barriers to movement.

Parking Farther...and Nutritious Movement

Through years of teaching folks, I (Katy) have found that the way we think about exercise is important when it comes to getting the movement we want and need. I use a "movement as nutrition" model.

There is no doubt movement nourishes our bodies. We need a certain amount of movement (think "movement minutes") most days, the same way we need calories from food, and there are movement macronutrients and movement micronutrients too. Different tissues and parts of the body are "fed" through movement, so our movement diet needs to be varied—just like we have to eat a wide range of foods to get all our dietary nutrients. This is good news! There are so many ways of moving that give our bodies what they need, it's super doable to find movement you enjoy and that fits into your life.

Humans have always needed to move, but in recent times, many activities of daily living have become so sedentary that we've begun to struggle to fit movement into our daily lives. This is a relatively new problem. Our grandparents and certainly their grandparents were not talking about exercise; the concept didn't really exist like it does now. We are part of one of the very first generations of people ever, in the history of humanity, to have even had to consider supplementing our lives with movement—movement has always been completely intertwined with everything a human has to do to survive, from gathering food to building shelter to holding infants on long walks.

This problem is so new and so huge that it's no wonder each of us struggles to figure out how to move enough. There are entire industries and fields of scientific study and governmental agencies devoted to this issue, and not a single one has gotten us all moving yet. Don't blame yourself for a systemic, culture-wide problem—but know that you can discover solutions, and tailor them to your specific life, to bring back your movement and all the health and joy that can come with it.

Advice like "park farther away from the store" is general and maybe even joyless on the surface, but it's an attempt, by all those scientists and governmental agencies, to make movement easier and more inclusive.

Just about everyone has to go to the store anyway, and you can fit in that movement right here, right now…nothing else needed. It's also a good reminder that not all movement needs to be exercise—you don't always need a period of time away from your day-to-day tasks, a special outfit, or even a specific fitness-y activity to move more (a lot more on this throughout the book!). We simply need to do more body-powered activity to balance out this new amount of sedentarism. So the parking advice is meant to show us that those movements are available to all of us, but part of the reason no one really takes it is *because* it's so general. To use this advice, we need to tailor it to our own bodies and lives.

Here's how you might harness the intention behind "park farther" advice to work for you and apply psychological flexibility along the way (the processes are *italicized*):

"Walking through the parking lot is boring." How about taking a *different perspective* and gamifying it? Walk on the curbs of a parking lot to challenge your balance, and now you're getting a dose of play (as well as more complex movement).

"I want to get this store chore done fast. My kid is here with me and I need to go figure out something to do with them." Remember your *values* and look at the five minutes in the lot as a way to connect. Obviously minding your safety, take a parking-lot lap together, jump over the cracks and painted lines, wonder at how grass can poke up through the concrete, or count the blue cars.

"I don't have three extra minutes." Great! Park farther away and don't take three extra minutes. *Accept* the challenge (and the discomfort that comes with it) and let your lack of time get you walking faster than you normally would (which is something we need to practice as we get older anyhow!).

"I forgot, and now I'm already parked close!" Cool, no problem; there are heaps of ways to get more movement. *Get present*, look around for other opportunities to move, and once inside the store, grab a basket instead of a cart, and let your arms schlep your load up and down the aisles. Look, you just got more movement…no parking farther required today.

See what you're learning to do here? You're becoming more flexible about how the "park farther" advice can apply to you in the moment, and you're finding a personalized solution to a giant, culture-wide problem.

You Helped Us Write This Book

We reached out to our communities and asked them to describe their personal barriers to movement, and a wide range of hurdles quickly came rolling in. We've loosely sorted the most common barriers into seven categories (some fall into more than one), then answered them one by one with our best psychological and human-movement insights. **You don't have to read this book straight through.** Feel free to jump (or flip, or hop) directly to the category or specific hurdle that most resonates with you.

1. I Am Not Motivated! (e.g., I don't care that exercise is good for me)
2. I Don't Have Enough Time! (e.g., I have too much work to do)
3. I Am So Embarrassed! (e.g., My thighs jiggle)
4. It's Uncomfortable! (e.g., It's too cold or too hot outside)
5. I'm Stuck on a Screen! (e.g., I'm addicted to my phone)
6. My Environment Makes It Impossible! (e.g., There are no sidewalks)
7. Other People Won't Move With Me! (e.g., My teenagers won't move)

Write it down

Barriers to movement are as diverse as the people who have them. That's why we wrote this book. Instead of writing yet another Top Ten Tips to Move More, or berating you for not making yourself exercise, we are offering a framework of psychological flexibility and a new way of looking at movement that you can apply to any movement barrier that shows up, including what might be the biggest barrier of all—being hard on yourself.

Embedded in every answer is the encouragement to approach your movement barriers with kindness and understanding. You can apply this methodology to a grocery store parking lot, but you can also apply it to your workplace, while spending time with people you love, and even in times when life gets stressful and your motivation wanes.

Before you get started, grab a blank notebook, and under the header *My Movement Barriers* jot down some of your personal reasons for not moving more. Keep this notebook with you as you read to apply this framework to your unique challenges! We will be asking you to answer questions, track a few things, and personalize everything you read here to your life.

The following pages address forty-four specific barriers. For each, you'll watch me (Diana) apply the processes of psychological flexibility that work best for that type of barrier. I (Katy) will be offering a different way to think about movement as well as some of the movement science and practical movement tips for the example. By looking at the way we do this again and again, you'll become more practiced in the steps, and soon you'll be able to work through your own barriers too.

To make it easier to follow and see the big picture, we have identified these processes with icons so that you can apply the framework for yourself.

We Can't Force It, and We Don't Have To

There's a lesson I (Diana) have learned from thousands of hours coaching people in behavior change: Trying to *make* yourself do something not only requires a lot of effort, it's also missing the big picture. If you are having a hard time moving your body, you are not alone. It makes perfect sense—our environments make it difficult to move and our psychology is such that we evolved to avoid uncomfortable things.

This book will offer you a solution that works far better than forcing yourself to exercise—it helps you understand the deeper psychological reasons you aren't moving the way you want, and it gives you the skills to address them. With the powerful processes of psychological flexibility and a fresh way of looking at exercise, you'll be able to transform your "I should exercise" into a motivation that comes from inside. And you'll finally be able to develop a sustainable movement practice that fits your life.

Here we go!

I'm Not Motivated

Motivation has to do with how much you want to do something, and in the upcoming reasons to avoid exercise, you'll see it comes in three different flavors: pleasure/excitement, avoiding unpleasant experiences, and connecting to values.

Pleasure- or excitement-driven motivation gives you the feeling of an upsurge of energy. It's a craving to do something because it feels good or exciting. Many of us are motivated to move because of the feeling it gives us; whether it's enjoying a sport, dancing with friends, or walking in nature, moving can feel good, fun, and joyous! It also releases chemicals into our body and brain that give us that feel-good buzz (endocannabinoids) and a feeling of focus and calm (serotonin), and make us want to keep doing it (dopamine). However, research suggests it can take about twenty minutes for these chemical systems to kick in, and if we haven't been active in a while, it can take a few *weeks* before moving starts to feel rewarding. Psychological flexibility processes can actually help you enjoy motivation more by getting present and savoring the pleasurable aspects of it.

The motivation to escape unpleasant experiences is often a big part of avoiding exercise. Many people are motivated to choose NOT to move, especially if they feel it is boring or uncomfortable, or that it brings back bad memories. As one of our readers said flat out, "I hate to sweat. As in, I *loathe it.*" As you will read in our solutions, applying psychological flexibility processes like acceptance, cognitive flexibility, and committed action can help a lot when we want to avoid movement because we find it unpleasant.

Both of these first two types of motivation—towards pleasure and away from pain—fluctuate day to day, affected by mood, expectations, energy levels, intensity of movement, and much more. You can't really create a long-term, sustainable movement plan based solely on whether you "feel like it" or "want to" do it, because it's too easily derailed by a motivation to avoid unpleasantness. What we need to get up and moving is something else—something deeper.

Values-Driven Motivation

The third flavor of motivation comes from your values. You can use your values as a kind of reservoir of deep motivation you can draw from whether or not you "want to" move.

Many of the reasons people cite for not moving have to do with lacking this third type of motivation. You'll see in our readers' barriers phrases like "I don't care if movement is good for me" or "I can't stick with it." Some of the barriers in this chapter might not even seem like they're about motivation at all (what does your dad making you do burpees when you were a kid have to do with motivation?), but if you drill down further, you'll see that underneath most of these reasons to not move is a disconnection from a deeper "movement why." Instead of waiting for your motivation to strike, you can turn to your values—what you care about most—as your inner motivator. You'll find that movement will support you in becoming more of the person you want to be, and also that when you bring your values to your movement, it becomes more meaningful.

Reason 1: I don't care that exercise is good for me, I just don't want to do it.

It sounds like knowing "exercise is good for you" isn't motivating for you. And really, it's not just you. Pretty much everyone knows that exercise is good for us, but very few of us want to do it. Only 25 percent of Americans meet the Centers for Disease Control and Prevention (CDC) minimum guidelines of 150 minutes of aerobic activity plus two days of strength training per week.

Let's be real: **If the data on exercise hasn't motivated you yet, it never will.** We need to figure out a deeper, more personal, and more intrinsic reason to move than "it's good for me." We're going to be talking a lot about values in this book, and it's super important for all of us in general to understand our values, so that we can stay connected with them and make sure we're living a life that aligns with the things we really care about.

So, heads up: This first barrier has a very long solution from us, because figuring out your values takes a bit of work and we want to make sure you understand it. This section will be useful whenever knowing your values is important to finding your way forward.

Core Values

Values are chosen by you, and they guide how you want to be in the world. They're characteristics/qualities you aspire to live by. Your values demonstrate what you care most about and how you express that care with your actions. To start exploring yours, get out your notebook and answer these questions:

- Choose a few parts of your life, what we'll call "domains," that are important to you (e.g., work, family, spirituality, friendship, leisure, community). How do you want to "show

15

up," or behave in them? For example, do you value being a fun parent? Being creative at work?

- In challenging situations, what principles do you want to guide your actions? How do you want to be when life gets hard? For example, do you want to be resilient, courageous, or determined? Or maybe flexible, creative, or accepting?

- What is the most meaningful part of your day? Is it when you're collaborating with others? Or maybe when you feel challenged and like you are growing stronger? Or is it when you are connecting with nature? What do these moments tell you about what you value?

Now let's drill down into your values a bit more. Use the following list (find an even longer list at uphill-books.com/IKISresources) to help you identify three values that stand out to you as really important. Your own values might not be listed here; this is just to give you some examples. Notice when you read the description of these values, they all come with an action. Values come to life when you demonstrate them with your behavior.

If you've never thought about your values this explicitly before, it might feel impossible to figure out which three are most important, and maybe you'll be hesitant to leave some important ones out! There's no FOMO in choosing values; you can live many of them throughout your day and life. Right now we're just helping you focus on a few you can use as guiding principles in your movement. Feel free to just choose three that resonate with you right now, and refer back to them throughout the book. If you find you're still not completely motivated or that they're not enough of a reason to get moving, revisit the list and see if there's something else that feels more important.

Do any of these resonate with you?

- Adventure: Embracing opportunities for new experiences and challenges.

- Collaboration: Joining forces with others to accomplish shared objectives.
- Compassion: Demonstrating empathy and actively working to alleviate suffering in oneself and others.
- Body awareness: Engaging in activities that deepen understanding and connection with your body.
- Nature connection: Spending time in nature and caring for the environment.
- Equity: Championing fairness and justice in all areas of life.
- Playfulness: Engaging in activities that bring joy, fun, and rejuvenation.
- Autonomy: Making choices that reflect independence and self-direction.
- Integrity: Living with honesty and staying true to your principles.
- Kindness: Acting with care and consideration towards others.
- Environmental stewardship: Making sustainable choices to protect the planet.

Once you've chosen a few core values, consider how movement impacts your ability to live out these values. For example, if tolerance is really important to you, does exercising on a regular basis help you to be more tolerant with your family or coworkers? Or if freedom is a core value, does doing your physical therapy exercises every day allow you more freedom to do some of the activities you love? Answer some of these questions in your notebook:

- How would moving your body more help you live out your values in the important domains of your life?
- How would moving your body more help you meet life's challenges in a way that you would feel proud of?

- How would moving your body more make your day more meaningful?

These all could be better reasons for you to move than "exercise is good for you." Values offer you a deeper intrinsic motivation. When you are *intrinsically* motivated to do something, you experience feelings of personal accomplishment and satisfaction that don't depend on an external source or outcome separate from the activity itself. Exercising because your doctor, your spouse, or an Instagram influencer tells you it's good for you is an extrinsic motivation. Sticking with a movement habit because it helps you be a more present partner or more resilient under stress, and those are things you value, is an intrinsic one.

Once you've taken a look at how your movement can support you in living out your personal values, let's see how you can also apply these values to how you move.

Take that list of three core values again. How could you demonstrate those values through moving your body? Here are some examples to get you started.

If you value personal growth, use movement as a way to challenge yourself and learn new skills.

If you value mindfulness, choose activities like yoga, tai chi, or a walk in nature to cultivate presence and awareness.

If you value collaboration, choose activities like sports, physical labor, or dance where you move with others.

If you value environmental stewardship, choose active transportation (walking or riding a bike to work).

If you value service/volunteering, find ways to move that help others, like joining a walk for charity, helping a friend move, or shoveling snow for your neighbor.

Get creative and see how many ways you can use your body to show what you care about.

Even if you don't care about exercising being good for you, there are a lot of things you do care about. When you link your values to movement, you'll not only be more motivated to do it, you'll also find that tending to your body with movement can make it easier to do what you love. Once you make the connection between moving your body more and how it impacts the important domains of your life in positive ways, you are likely to feel more intrinsically motivated to move. If you're sitting by the back door with your running shoes laced but part of you just wants to go crawl back into bed, you can call on your core values to get yourself out the door. If one of your core values is connection, and movement makes you a more present dad, remind yourself of that. If you one of your core values is productivity, and movement makes you more alert and creative, remind yourself of that. What you personally care about is what will always be the most motivating to you.

Rethinking Movement
Find Your "Core Moves"

Just as you're getting more specific with your values around movement, you can get more specific about the movements that go into the activities you value. Think about the physical shape of the actions and activities that make your life meaningful. For example, if you value service and want to participate in a community garden or work at the local foodbank, consider the movements those acts of service are made of: unloading and stacking boxes, squatting and bending the spine, dragging heavy bags, etc.

If you value independence, i.e., "being able to meet your own needs," think about what that value means physically to you now and into the future too. Be as specific as you can. Does this mean things like balance, grip strength, knees and/or hips free from pain, the ability to drive (turning the neck and shoulders well)?

If you value nature connection, get clear on the movements that facilitate this for you. Is it a long walk outside? Setting up a tent? Sitting on a blanket beneath a tree?

List the movements that are important to the tasks you identify (like sitting cross-legged on the ground; walking three, five, or ten miles; having shoulder mobility). Once you've got a list of the body movements needed for your meaningful moves, look to see which movements show up over and over again. Just as you identified three or four core values, take the time to identify your three or four "core movements" and write them down! My (Katy) personal core moves are walking, squatting, and hanging from a bar. Life gets busy, but when I dedicate a little bit of time to each of these most days (at least thirty minutes to walking, and my squatting and hanging practice are less than ten minutes total, and no, I don't do all of these movements at once), I can show up for all other areas of my life without my body feeling like it's working against me.

Your core moves might be "stretch out on the floor once a day, pick up something that weighs twenty pounds, and take a flight of stairs." Or, "bend over to touch my toes, walk with a backpack, and jump." Like values, there's no right set—the things you value and the activities that are meaningful to you are defined only by you. These movements are valuable to you, dear reader, because they're conduits to your values, and fitting their practice in isn't important because the movements are "good for you," but because they facilitate experiences that give your life meaning.

Reason 2: Exercise is uncomfortable; I hate sweating. As in loathe it.

I (Katy) am going to jump in right up top to say that there are plenty of ways of moving that nourish your body that don't involve sweat. But because there are many ways of moving that nourish your body that *do* leave you sweaty, let's address your sweat-hatred first, then we'll get back to changing the way we think about movement.

I (Diana) am wondering two things: How did hating to sweat develop for you, and does your aversion to sweating impact your life in other ways beyond exercise?

Aversions

When we have a strong aversion to something, it might be just a personal sensitivity or preference. For example, I hate sour cream (as in I *loathe* it) and I always have. But our fears and aversions can also come from negative experiences. Maybe you began to hate sweating in seventh grade when someone teased you for sweaty armpits, or your big sister told you that sweating was gross, or maybe like many of us, you were influenced by media telling you that natural body functions are something to cover up, hide, or get rid of by buying this product.

Exploring the origins of your loathing can help loosen up this block to exercise. Grab your notebook and answer these questions about sweating (and note, dear reader, you can do this for other things you loathe too!):

- When did your aversion to sweating first show up for you? Was it linked to a negative experience? What do you remember feeling emotionally and physically during that time?

- What messages have you received about sweating from your family, your friends, the media? Are they linked to personal characteristics such as being unfeminine, smelly, having poor hygiene, or something else?

- Does your loathing get stronger in some situations than others—e.g., social situations, under stress, at work, times when you are being evaluated or in the spotlight?

Knowing the roots of your aversion won't necessarily change your behavior, but it can help you step back and see what's happening for you with more perspective. Maybe you can develop self-compassion; it's hard to hate something your body naturally does. Remember, self-compassion is treating yourself and your body with the same care you would a good friend, a child, or even a stranger. All bodies sweat, make weird noises, get injured, get old, ache now and then, and change over time. If we hate the natural processes of our body, we end up in a battle with nature! You may not enjoy all of your bodily processes (trust us, hot flashes are not fun), but you can be understanding about it. Would you tell a teenager that they should *loathe* their pimples, or your mom that she should *loathe* her wrinkles? Of course not. It's all par for the course of having a human body.

Missing Out On Life

As stated before, trying to avoid unpleasant experiences is a big motivator for *not* exercising. Our next question is this: Is avoiding things that make you sweat narrowing your life in other ways?

Avoidance of discomfort can really limit our ability to move freely and fully in our lives. Sure, in the short term we don't have to feel that uncomfortable sensation or feeling, but in the long term we miss out on things that may be important to us. Our fear chooses for us, before we even get a chance to decide if it's something we want to do or not. For example, if you loathe sweating, you may avoid getting up at a wedding and dancing, playing ball with your dog, heading to the beach on a hot summer day with friends, or taking that trek to Machu Picchu you've always wanted to take. And, the more you avoid your fears, the stronger they tend to get! Plus, you never grow the confidence to handle your discomfort, and you avoid any chances for contradictory evidence to prove your fears wrong. Consider these questions for yourself:

- What are all the things you avoid because you might sweat—activities, occasions, events, etc.? Make a list.
- Are any of these things linked to your values?
- When you avoid these things, does it make you feel less or more confident you can handle sweating?

Ultimately, avoiding discomfort and resisting reality narrows our life and makes things worse. So, what can we do when we really don't like something, but avoiding it is getting in the way of the movement we want? Practice *acceptance*.

Forcing and Accepting Are Different

Getting more comfortable with being uncomfortable is actually a skill you can develop and strengthen, but there's a catch: Don't force it! Forcing yourself to do things you hate makes you hate them even more (especially if you are muttering to yourself the whole time, "I loathe this!"). Acceptance has more to do with opening up to and allowing for some discomfort as you take actions towards your values. If the word *acceptance* rubs you the wrong way, try on other words and phrases that mean the same thing:

- allow
- let go
- open up
- let it be
- it is what it is
- be with

You're in a game of tug-of-war with your discomfort around sweating, and not sweating is winning. Acceptance is like letting go of the rope. Once you stop playing tug-of-war, you free up energy to do things that you care about.

Research shows that people who practice acceptance of difficult thoughts and feelings during exercise, as opposed to trying to suppress them, are more likely to be successful at maintaining their exercise habit. But getting better at accepting takes practice! Here are some ways you can practice acceptance to increase your openness to sweat.

Accept the sweat...with your mind: Next time you exercise or move your body in a way that makes you sweat, spend the first two minutes saying in your mind, "I loathe this." Really get into it. Loathe sweating with all your might. Notice what happens. Do you hate it even more? Does it make it even harder? Or maybe after one minute you just think you are being ridiculous. Then, turn your mental energy around. Spend the next few minutes saying to yourself, "I am open to this. I allow this. It is what it is." Or, even simpler, just say "Yes" with every step you take. What happens? Does it change how you relate to your sweating when you accept it?

Accept the sweat...with your body: Choose an activity where you might sweat and embody a posture of acceptance while you do it. Notice if you are gripping, tensing up, or resisting with your body. Where can you loosen your hold a little? Can you relax your face? Release your jaw? Exhale? Soften your gaze? Unclench your hands? Lower your shoulders? When you let go with your body, you send a signal to your brain that you are safe. Sure it's uncomfortable, but sweating is not physically harming you.

Build Your Acceptance Muscle

If you want to get better at accepting the discomfort of sweat, you can also practice accepting the discomfort of other things that you feel uncomfortable with. Evidence suggests that intentionally stepping outside your comfort zone—a concept known as *behavioral stretching*—can enhance your wellbeing. Every time you prove to yourself that you can handle discomfort, you get a little more confident. Challenging situations feel less daunting, and when you experience success it creates a positive feedback loop. Plus, doing things outside your comfort zone brings a freshness and newness to life—it breaks you out of your routine, which can feel invigorating. Practice some behavioral stretching by engaging in activities that make you physically uncomfortable on purpose (they don't have to be related to sweating). You could try walking barefoot, learning a complicated move or dance routine from TikTok, or getting up an hour earlier for a week.

Try at least one thing—anything!—outside your comfort zone this week, and as you do it, remember you are building your acceptance muscle.

Good stressors

Strengthening your acceptance muscle isn't just about your psychology—it can be good for your biology too. Hormesis is the process of exposing your body to something that at a high dose would be damaging, but at a (usually intermittent) lower dose causes you to adapt in a positive way. Hormetic stressors include things like short, intense bouts of exercise (think sprinting), cold plunges, or intermittent fasting. This type of moderate, intermittent exposure builds up what Dr. Elissa Epel, author of *The Stress Prescription*, calls your stress resilience.

In addition to other benefits, these types of physical stressors increase your body's ability to handle stress. Yes, you're uncomfortable, but only for a short period of time, and your body gets better at physically recovering quickly. Psychologically, these types of hormetic stressors are also a great way to work out and strengthen your "acceptance muscle." Let go, open up, and be willing to accept the discomfort that comes with a dunk in a cold river or a quick sprint up a few flights of stairs. Your body is building stress resilience.

The most successful motivation to move is our values. Right now the discomfort sweat is creating for your body and mind is your source of motivation, and you're being directed away from exercise because of it. Even though you loathe sweating, your loathing of it doesn't have to run your life. You are in charge, not your sweat! By accepting with your mind, body, and behavior, you will be able to open up, little by little, to experiences that make you sweat, but more importantly you'll open up to ways of moving in the world that align with what you care about!

Was sweating really that bad?

We're not the best at predicting how tough something will be, especially when it comes to exercise. Research shows that people generally expect workouts to be less pleasant and more exhausting than they actually are, a phenomenon called *affective forecasting error*. This habit of underestimating how enjoyable physical activity can be often messes with our motivation. Interestingly, the more inactive you are, the more likely you are to assume exercise will be unpleasant—yet both active and inactive people tend to enjoy it equally. In this case, our minds aren't exactly trustworthy.

Despite our anticipation of it, once we start exercising, it is often more enjoyable than we predicted. Just as our bodies evolved to preserve energy, so too did they evolve to move—to get resources, protect us from threats, find a mate, and socially connect through play. That's why, once you get going, it starts to feel good. Your body releases neurohormones like dopamine and endorphins that can make movement more enjoyable than your tricky mind predicted.

Rethinking Movement
Why We Sweat (And When We Don't Need To)

Before I (Katy) get to the ways you can move that don't make you sweat, here's *why* bodies sweat: With the exception of a genetic mutation that makes you sweat a lot, all the time, sweat is all about cooling us down. Bodies are heavy objects, and moving our parts around takes effort. The work of moving (muscles contracting to move your bony levers) can heat you up, and your body sweats to keep from overheating.

If you've got a type of movement you love, you can sweat less by getting more flexible in how you approach it: pick a cooler time of day, add a fan, drink cool water, wear clothes that breathe and trap less heat, go for a shorter duration.

I mentioned before, there are plenty of movements your body needs that don't require sweat. Find a modality of movement that doesn't heat you up as much: a long slow walk, an hour of stretching, or an easygoing bike ride can be good options when you're shying away from sweat.

Your body *should* sweat now and then—the practice of sweating is what keeps up your body's ability to do so, which is crucial—but while you're practicing becoming more tolerant over time, you can choose to move in ways that don't leave you sticky.

Reason 3: Exercise feels monotonous and boring, and it's the last thing I want to do with my free time.

It's hard to drum up motivation when you think something is boring, Nobody wants to spend their free time doing monotonous and tedious tasks!

So, how can we make movement less tedious and more enjoyable—something you look forward to? Two psychological tools can help with changing our perspective: temptation bundling and savoring. Let's unpack each to transform "Exercise is boring" into "I'm motivated to do this!"

Temptation Bundling

Exercise can often feel more like a "should" than a want. You know it's good for you in the long term, but you don't want to invest the time *right now*. Temptation bundling is pairing something that has delayed rewards (exercise, in this case) with something that is pleasurable in the short term. In a large research study with over six thousand participants, when subjects were told to pair their session with a pleasurable audiobook they only listened to when they exercised, it boosted their likelihood of doing a weekly workout by 10–14 percent. Why? When you temptation bundle exercise, it's instantly less boring and more gratifying.

Being with friends can turn into a pickleball meetup. Your love for coffee can turn into a walk to the local café to grab a cup. Stretching your hips or being active in the garden can pair nicely with listening to your favorite podcast.

To shift your perspective on exercise monotony, think about the type of exercise you're trying to motivate yourself to do, then come up with some fun, enjoyable activities you can do or environments you can create at the same time. You can try some of these ideas:

- Take a walk at the farmers' market.
- Call your sister while walking.
- Watch your favorite show at the gym (and only at the gym!).
- Wear your most comfy exercise clothes while you move.
- Bike along the prettiest streets.
- Book a class with your favorite instructor.

I (Diana) temptation bundle by stretching while watching our favorite family show, *The Amazing Race*. Teams are racing around the world, and I send my foot around in circles, or take a figure four stretch to work on my hips, or practice doing headstands with my kids. My body thanks me for it, and it feels better to move while watching people sprint to the finish line.

I (Katy) love rocking out to music, but between work and family time, I struggle to find time to blast what I want to hear. So for me, heading out for a walk is just as much about a chance to listen to music uninterrupted as it is the exercise of taking a walk. Looking forward to picking out my own music is often what motivates me at the end of the day.

With temptation bundling, it's pretty simple: to make your movement less monotonous, pair it with something else you love. And be present while you do it (don't worry, we're about to teach you how!).

Savoring

You can also make movement less boring by bringing awareness to the full experience of moving your body...and savoring it. *Savoring* is the act of intentionally paying attention to, appreciating, and enhancing the positive aspects of an experience. When you savor your experience, it increases your positive emotions, helps with stress reduction, and can turn even the most mundane experiences into pleasurable ones.

The key here is to be fully present with pleasurable aspects of what you are doing—flexibly shining your attention spotlight on the good stuff. This doesn't mean ignoring discomfort; it's more about attentional shift—which involves the psychological flexibility processes of perspective-taking and being present. You get to choose where you place your attention.

Try this right now: Let your chin drop towards your chest, then gently bring your right ear towards your right shoulder, then slowly take your left ear to your left shoulder. Where is the movement restricted? Where is it easy? Linger on the spots that could use a little extra love. Breathe into and around the areas that are tight and relax your shoulders. Close your eyes and luxuriate in the chance to rest your mind as you roll. Have gratitude for this moment to be with your body. Even the most monotonous things can become interesting when you are present for them and savor them.

There are five ways to savor an experience, according to Erika Miyakawa, a Japanese psychologist who researches savoring: thanksgiving, basking, marveling, luxuriating, and knowing. They all involve being fully present with your experience. Let's explore how you can apply each of these to your movement or exercise.

Pick a physical activity that you usually find tedious or repetitive (for me, Diana, this is walking in circles around the airport while waiting to board, or my son's baseball practice while he's doing drills). Now try to apply each of these types of savoring to it. Notice how it changes your experience.

Thanksgiving: Appreciate the opportunity to move your body. Feel gratitude for this chance to move. Appreciate the place, people, and activities you get to engage with by moving your body.

Basking: Take in feelings of pride at growing stronger in your body with movement. Feel the accomplishment of living out your values, finishing a challenging workout, or meeting movement goals.

Marveling: Let yourself feel awe through movement. Be amazed by the beauty of nature, surprising sights, and the capabilities of your human body.

Luxuriating: Enjoy the physical and sensory pleasures of movement. Enjoy the good feeling of stretching your muscles, the release of tension and stress, the flow of your body, or the creativity of movement.

Knowing: Savor the wisdom that comes through moving your body—the knowledge you gain from interacting with new places, fresh faces, experiences, and challenges, or the knowledge gained by learning about yourself and your capacities.

The next time you find exercise a drag, dear reader, try these two techniques: pair it with something that is enjoyable (temptation bundling) and focus your attention on the positive aspects of movement (savoring). The most important factor in both is being fully present—shifting your attention to here and now, and the good that can come with moving your body.

Rethinking Movement
Make It Playful

Exercise often has to be slotted into our free time, where it's competing with all the other things we enjoy doing. For many, exercise can feel like a chore: boring! Counting reps or laps, monitoring intensity, and paying attention to other metrics is the opposite of play, and when it comes to motivating ourselves to pick movement, we might need to boost the fun factor.

Any movement can become playful—play has more to do with your attitude than the specific activity—and playful activities can be easier to stick to. Sports and physical games, like pickleball and Kubb (a backyard throwing game) count, but it's also playful to get a weighted hoop going around your midsection for fifteen minutes while you're standing in the living room. Reroute your daily walk past a playground, where you can go across the monkey bars, ride the slide, and hop on the swings to challenge your vestibular/balance system. Put on your favorite dance music and boogie. I (Diana) keep a big open space in our living room solely for the purpose of fun movement. Over the years we've played balloon volleyball and Twister, and made forts together there. Open spaces are great invitations for the whole family to move.

Think about the physical activities you loved as a kid, back before you thought about them being good for you and instead just thought they were fun. For me (Katy), some playful activities were "being a mermaid" in the pool for hours, riding bikes with my sister around our neighborhood until dark, and hitting tennis balls against the side of the house by myself. When you're looking to add movement, there's no need to pick from a list of activities you find boring. Find exercise that closely resembles your "play" list so it's easier to choose.

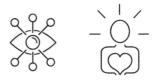

Reason 4: My dad pressured me to exercise as a kid. He was rigid about it and I still hate burpees to this day. I think I'm still rebelling in some way now by choosing not to move. I just don't want to.

We're sad you had to endure this experience as a kid. It's unacceptable for children to be coerced into physical activity or subjected to exercise as a form of punishment. It's also completely natural to have a rebellious response to something that caused you harm. However, not moving as an adult only ends up hurting you further.

Many of us had negative experiences with exercise and movement as kids. Whether it was being forced to take swimming lessons or climb the ropes in gym, being shamed or ridiculed for being slow or clumsy, or being left out of activities and sports because we weren't athletic enough, we all have stories about ourselves that we carry from our early experiences that can make us hesitant and unmotivated to move our bodies as adults.

Practice Self-Compassion

Although we cannot go back and change our early childhoods, we can change how we respond to ourselves now, as adults. Self-compassion is a powerful strategy that involves caring for yourself in the way you would care for someone else you love. Research shows that when you are compassionate towards yourself you are more likely to stay committed to your values during hard times, be more resilient, and have higher engagement with your goals. What's more, people with more self-compassion are more likely to be physically active, feel more confident that they can overcome barriers to movement, and have reduced psychological distress (such as anxiety and depression).

In the following visualization, you will get a chance to develop your own inner compassionate parent, one that can care for you now and support you in finding a kinder way to relate to movement.

A compassionate parent wants the best for you, is attuned to your emotions and physical needs, and is encouraging, engaged, and wise. They pay attention to and respond to your cues with understanding and support. One way to do this for yourself is to use compassionate perspective-taking, to start seeing yourself and tending to yourself the way a compassionate parent would. Start with the steps below. You can either visualize this exercise, or get our your notebook and write some of your answers down. You can also find an audio version of this exercise on our resource page, uphill-books.com/IKISresources, if that works better for you.

1. Take three long, slow, soothing breaths. Slowing your breathing down in this way will settle your nervous system and help you make contact with the most compassionate version of yourself. Take your time with this. If you need more than three breaths to settle, take more. And if slow breathing doesn't do it for you, try a simple relaxation exercise where you let go of any gripping in your face, your shoulders, your belly, your hips, and your feet. When you feel more at ease, continue to the next step.

2. Think back to your childhood when you had a negative experience with exercise. Tune in to your feelings at that time. What was it like for you? What was hard for you? What would you have wanted to tell someone, if you could?

3. Now imagine you could go back in time and meet yourself as a kid. You are the compassionate parent that you needed back then. You are attuned, encouraging, engaged, and wise. What comforting words or touch would you offer yourself? Would you want to give yourself a hug, or maybe just listen?

4. Knowing what you know now about movement and exercise, what would you want to tell your younger self? If you could offer yourself some supportive words, what would you say? What wisdom would you relay? What advice would you give about exercise and your body?

5. Now, take this compassionate adult into the present. If you were encouraging, attuned, wise, and caring towards yourself around movement now, what would you tell yourself? How would you move your body? What wisdom does this compassionate inner parent offer you now?

Choosing to move your body is one of the kindest things you can do for yourself—especially if you are choosing to move your body from a place of love. You can transform your past in the present moment by changing how you relate to yourself. A compassionate perspective offers a different way of relating to yourself and movement, and when you choose to parent yourself with compassion, you rebel in a different way. Rebel by offering yourself the understanding and care you didn't get around movement as a kid.

Reframing Movement
Rebel Movement

Exercise itself can be a rigid concept, but movement doesn't have to be fitness-y or feel like bootcamp to benefit the body. Good news, rebel! You're totally in charge of your exercise programming now, and if you want to have an exercise-free movement diet at this point, you totally can. All those burpees can go take a hike.

"Gym class trauma" and the like is very much a thing and folks have been working hard to change the culture of PE and sports so that they help connect people better to their bodies, not the opposite. Movement is rarely something we truly despise, because ultimately it makes our bodies feel so much better. You might just need movements that exist outside the fitness/athletic paradigm to start with—things that feel very different from your father's approach. Brainstorm ways of moving that feel the opposite of rigid as you start to explore ways of moving you actually enjoy and find meaningful. Only you can know for sure what would feel different; our role here is to let you know that *all* kinds of movement nourish your body, and that includes dancing in your kitchen, going on a coffee shop crawl by foot, putting your arms and hands to work in pottery class, and sitting on the ground cross-legged for a picnic. You might want entirely different modes of movement than you were forced to do, but you might also be okay with some exercises as long as you do them for the length of time or at the time of day that suits you. The key here is, you're in charge, rebel, and you get to tend to your body through movement in whatever way you want. So, what do you want to do?

Reason 5: I am great at starting exercise programs (give me a thirty-day program and I'll sign up!), but I can't seem to stick with them. I give up on day twenty-five and go back to my old way of doing things.

Guess what?! Thirty-day plans are the opposite of habit-forming; they come with their own expiration date (you never have to do this again in twenty-nine more days!). You are not alone, dear reader. About half of people who start an exercise program drop out within six months.

The most successful longtime exercisers have built movement into their daily life by making it a habit. When you make movement a habit, you are more likely to sustain it, even if your motivation is low. Consider habits like teeth brushing, saying thank you, making your bed, or handwashing. At first you probably needed to be reminded to do them, you had to practice them, and you needed to be rewarded for doing them (even if the reward was intrinsic—look at me! I tied my own shoes!). But over time, unlike thirty-day plans, habits take less effort to keep going because they become a way of life (although, depending on your life circumstances, sometimes these habits have to be re-learned again—like how we all learned how to wash our hands more diligently during the pandemic). But you can turn any movement you want into a daily habit, one that lasts longer than just thirty days.

Ride out the motivation wave. According to Stanford behavioral economist B. J. Fogg, motivation comes in waves. It sounds like when you sign up for your thirty-day program you have a temporary surge in motivation. However, motivation changes from day to day, and month to month. You are probably extra motivated to sign up for a thirty-day exercise program if it's January, or you have a wedding coming up, or a milestone birthday. But what happens when the program is over, your wedding is done, or you turn forty-one? Do you give up on exercise? The problem with thirty-day plans, or jumping onto big motivation waves, is that they don't support lasting change. You need a movement plan that taps into your deeper values (see Reason 1), is easy to do when your motivation is low, is simple when life gets complicated, and can adjust depending on your energy.

Get off the thirty-day bandwagon with its built-in message that this is going to end, and get into a lifelong, flexible commitment to movement. The what and how of exercise look different across life stages, but the commitment to keeping your values-based habit is unwavering.

Make it simple and small. To design a lasting movement habit, you need to explore which types of movement you can realistically add to your life. If you want a habit to be sustainable, you need to start small and make it doable. Humans tend to resist hard things, especially when our motivation wave is low. For example, I (Diana) wanted to add more yoga into my week but couldn't figure out how to fit in a yoga class after work. So instead, I started doing sun salutations in my ten-minute breaks between clients. By the end of the day I had accumulated about the same amount of active yoga as I would if I were at a class. Small movements, accumulated over the course of the day, are beneficial for physical health. Take a moment to brainstorm a big movement you want to add to your day, like "Walk four miles a day" or "Start strength training." Then, think about ways to break these down into small, specific, actionable behaviors (or you can call them "steps").

A behavior is an action, not a want or aspiration. "I want to move my body more" is not a behavior. But if your big movement goal is to walk four miles a day, small, simple behaviors could be "Walk twenty minutes around the neighborhood," "Do one errand on foot," and "Walk home from work on Fridays." If you want to start strength training, simple and small behaviors could be "Do counter push-ups while waiting for the kettle to boil," "Practice lunges during commercial breaks," and "Take the stairs two at a time."

Design your cues and rewards. Habits follow a predictable pattern: A cue triggers you to engage in the behavior (e.g., it's my ten-minute break between clients), you do the behavior (sun salutations), and then you experience a consequence that reinforces the behavior (I feel more focus and less back pain in my next session). Cues signal you to engage in the behavior and rewards, including intrinsic rewards, keep the behavior going.

So the next step in habit formation is picking a cue to signal you to engage in your simple, small movement behavior. It works best if you pick a cue that is already happening in your daily routine.

Here are some examples of cues that can signal behaviors:

- After I make coffee, I walk my dog.
- After I drop the kids off at school, I go to Pilates class.
- After I eat lunch, I go for a thirty-minute walk.
- After I turn on my favorite show, I get on the floor and stretch.

Complete this sentence for yourself and write it in your notebook: *After I _____, I will _____.*

Once you set up your cue for movement, add in a reward to keep your movement going. Rewards can include savoring the good feeling of movement (see page 29), reminding yourself of your values (see pages 15–19), or giving yourself a reward when you complete the movement. Complete this sentence and write it in your notebook: *When I _____, I will reward my behavior by _____.*

Make your habits flexible. After working with hundreds of people on behavior change, I've noticed the thing that throws people off the most: rigid beliefs about what constitutes success and failure. Maybe this sounds familiar: "I didn't get up in time to walk this morning; I'll skip it for today." Or this: "I went on vacation for two weeks; I can't get back on track with movement now." Believing that movement only counts if it's linear or uninterrupted guarantees you're going to fall off the wagon.

We all get sick, go on vacation, have busy days at work, get stuck in traffic, prioritize caretaking, or sleep past our alarms. A flexible habit is one that can adapt with you and withstand these types of normal life changes. Consider some of the habits you designed above. How will you get flexible with them when life throws you a curveball?

For example, there are a lot of ways I (Diana) build movement into what could traditionally be seen as sedentary work. Some days that's sitting on a ball during a session, writing my notes while stretching on the floor, or offering walking sessions to clients who have expressed they don't have time to squeeze movement and therapy and all the things into their day.

Make your movement a flexible habit and it can become a reliable part of your life, not just a thirty-day plan.

Rethinking Movement
Look For the Minutes

There's a misconception that movement only counts if it's a longer bout of exercise. But that's not true. For example, one study found that doing vigorous exercise for just under three minutes a day was linked to a 40 percent reduction in developing heart disease. Minutes matter!

You likely have a handful of unoccupied minutes every day, long enough to be detectable but too short a time to do any big activity, in which you can grow a new movement habit. First, you need to identify that bit of time when you're in it. I (Katy) find a little bit of free time shows up when I'm waiting, usually in a car, to pick up a kid. Maybe it's in the morning while you're waiting for your tea kettle to boil or your computer to boot up. Catching yourself in this space is key, because you're going to use the act of catching yourself as your cue to move.

Second, identify an action you will take whenever you catch your bit of free time. Maybe it's walking for five minutes, doing one or two shoulder stretches, or doing a balance challenge. Whatever your action of choice is, do that instead of hopping onto the phone for a scroll.

Once you're tuned in to spotting little pockets of downtime and have a plan ready to go whenever they pop up (likely more often than you realized), you'll be on your way to moving more every day. Thirty-day exercise programs are compelling because they hook us in with their low commitment. Capitalize on that same attraction—it's just a few minutes of exercise!—and let it help you build a habit that will serve you for years.

Reason 6: I've not exercised for so long, it's going to hurt too much to do it. I can't start again.

You are offering a glimpse here of what it must be like to be in your mind when you try to get started. Does it tell you things like *It's going to hurt too much* or *I can't start again?* Our mind has a tendency to amplify the negative and remind us a lot that things are going to hurt.

But, you might be thinking, *it is going to hurt!* Before we debate that, try to notice that that is your mind talking. You have thoughts, commentary, images popping into your mind all day long. Some of these thoughts are helpful to your movement motivation, and some derail you. If I (Diana) were to listen to my mind's stories while writing this book for you (*am I doing a good job? Is this making sense? I'm boring them*), I wouldn't get many words on the page.

Noticing your mind is a skill. In Acceptance and Commitment Therapy (ACT), we call this cognitive flexibility. The idea behind cognitive flexibility is that you can't get rid of thoughts, but you can be aware of your own thinking, thereby getting separation from those thoughts. If you are wondering, *Who is noticing my mind, if it's not my mind? Or is it my mind noticing itself?* then you're asking a great question.

When you realize, *Oh, I'm having that same old thought that I'm too tired to walk*, you're relating differently to the times you believe that statement at face value—"I'm too tired to walk." So, then, who is noticing your mind? It's actually your mind, observing your own *thinking*. It's not really about a separate "mind"; it's a part of you watching your thoughts without being fully engrossed in them—kind of like having an internal observer.

When you use this internal observer, and see that a thought is just a thought—much like a movie on a screen—you will feel that your thoughts have less power over you. Cognitive flexibility allows you to choose whether you want to listen to a thought or not. We don't always have to just follow our mind's advice, especially when it doesn't align with our values-based goals. You can observe thoughts, evaluate their helpfulness, and then let them go or act on them depending on what works best for you (that wise observer self). The fact is, the thoughts streaming continuously through your mind throughout the day aren't all helpful, and just because you have a thought doesn't mean you have to act on it. For example, you might say in your mind right now, *I can't stand up. I can't stand up. I can't stand up.* But even as you say this, you can still stand up (or raise your hand, blink your eyes, smile, depending on your body's ability). Having a thought doesn't necessarily make it true (and sometimes your thoughts are true, but still not helpful).

Take a moment to consider all of the demotivating things your mind tells you about exercise and physical activity (true or not!). Read through this list, and notice how when you believe these thoughts it impacts your motivation to exercise:

- It's going to hurt too much.
- I am out of shape.
- This is too hard.
- I can't start exercising again.
- It's too early in the morning to exercise.

When you attach on to and follow these thoughts, what happens?

Now try this. Repeat these thoughts, but add the disclaimer "I'm having the thought that":

- I'm having the thought that it's going to hurt too much.
- I'm having the thought that I am out of shape.
- I'm having the thought that this is too hard.
- I'm having the thought that I can't start again.
- I'm having the thought that it's too early.

Practicing cognitive flexibility involves noticing that a thought is just a thought and it doesn't have to determine your behavior.

Choosing Compassionate Thoughts

Another practice that may be helpful to you when these demotivating thoughts show up is to choose a more helpful thought, a self-compassionate one.

Self-compassion isn't letting yourself off the hook; rather, it's reminding yourself that it's human to get off track from your values, and using kindness to gently guide yourself back.

Self-compassion involves recognizing that you are struggling, and offering yourself support to help minimize your suffering.

According to self-compassion researcher Kristin Neff, self-compassion has both a tender (yin) side and an active, fierce (yang) side. The tender side of compassion is soft, kind, warm, and loving towards you when you feel guilty about not exercising. The fierce side of self-compassion is protective, active, and brave enough to do something about it.

What are some warm, encouraging, and courageous thoughts you might choose to tell yourself when you're getting started? Can you link your compassionate thoughts to your values? Write them in your notebook under the title *Compassionate Thoughts*. Your compassionate thoughts might look something like this:

- It's understandable this is hard; it's often hard to get started again.
- I love adventure, and getting back in shape will help me do what I love.
- I've been able to do this before, and I know I can do it again.
- I can take it slow and be gentle with myself.
- I am doing this to care for myself, and sometimes caring for myself is uncomfortable.
- Every time I start again I grow stronger and more resilient.

As you get started again with moving your body, remember to notice your thoughts, be flexible with the ones that are unhelpful and demotivating (*I am having the thought that…*), and choose compassionate thoughts that are warm and encouraging.

By practicing these skills of cognitive flexibility and self-compassion, you can and will get moving again, no matter what your mind says.

Rethinking Movement
Why Does Exercise Hurt?

When I (Katy) was in college, I was trying to start a regular exercise habit and decided to sign up for my first group exercise class at the gym: 6:00 a.m. strength-training sessions, Monday, Wednesday, and Friday. The instructor was a great teacher—inspiring and gave lots of coaching on good form. The very first session ended with walking lunges while holding weights. (If you've never done this move, it's a booty killer.) I had never done a walking lunge, let alone enough to fill ten minutes, but the instructor was using eight-pound weights so I grabbed those too and did every lunge she did. She was a very motivating teacher! When I woke up the next morning, I felt like I had been in an accident. I could barely get out of bed, and when I did, I couldn't walk right. Every step felt like a giant punch to my thighs. The soreness went away after a few days, but needless to say, I didn't make it to any more exercise classes that week.

The soreness that comes with exercise is most often related to tissue damage—tiny microtears in worked muscles and connective tissue, as a result of dealing with a new load. This damage is the whole point of exercise. By doing movements we're not used to, or while carrying more weight or moving for longer than we usually do, we create microdamage that the body responds to by growing more mass. The process of healing and getting stronger includes a little inflammation and swelling, which can make the body painful to the touch, and cause stiffness and soreness too. Unless you're like me, and you jump headfirst into a session that is way too much of a workout to start with, exercise-related soreness is fairly mild, lasting a day or two.

Just as there are many exercises that don't make you sweat, there are a lot that won't make you sore, either. Pace yourself; start with shorter sessions and try things without much weight or impact at first. Do a little bit every day as opposed to a lot on just one or two days a week, until you've felt things out.

If you feel your pain from exercise is due to a bigger injury being created by the way you're exercising, then getting assistance with form or some physical therapy on a weak area might be a good place to start. While exercise does leave you a bit sore in general, especially when you're just getting started, your workout shouldn't leave you in regular pain. Stop and sort out some of the holes in your movements by working on corrective exercise part-by-part until you can move with relative ease.

Reason 7: I used to have a really unhealthy relationship with movement. I would go to the gym and run on the treadmill for hours, exercise even if I was sick, and skip out on social stuff to get my workout in. I don't exercise now because I'm afraid my obsessive self will take over. Exercise is not my friend.

Hey! How did my personal barrier get in here? I (Diana) am in recovery from a longtime struggle with compulsive exercise (along with anorexia, bulimia, and binge eating). For decades I used exercise to control my weight, compensate for overeating, and avoid feeling difficult emotions. I obsessively exercised to feel a sense of control, only to find that exercise controlled me. Exercise took over my life, and my relationship with my body became a mechanistic one. Instead of enjoying movement, movement became a "have to" and no longer a choice. It's been a long, slow process to get to the point where movement is my friend again. But it is possible. Where exercise once was isolating and rigid for me, it is now connecting, creative, and restorative.

Many people recovering from unhealthy relationships with exercise fear it. If you have a history of disordered exercise, you might have an all-or-nothing mindset when it comes to movement. Or you may not be motivated to move because you fear you'll push yourself too far, get obsessive, or use exercise as punishment. Here's a few things I do, and that I coach my clients to do, to make friends with movement again.

Ditch the calorie and step counters. Self-monitoring is a very effective strategy in behavior change. Just the act of measuring something is likely to change your behavior (for better or worse!). Given that, it's wise to choose what you are tracking carefully. If you are measuring calories burned, you are likely to become more preoccupied with calories. If you are measuring steps made, you just might find yourself walking in circles around your living room to get to ten thousand. There's nothing wrong with these measurements, but if you find yourself becoming obsessed with these numbers or that they make you rigid, they may not be the best things for you to track.

Maybe you'll need to ditch the programs, apps, and devices that count your calories, steps, or miles, and avoid machines that ask for your weight or measure your progress in numbers. You may be able to use those again in the future, but in the beginning they can be deterrents from tuning in to what feels good to your body. Choose different ways to track your progress, such as asking yourself:

- How does exercise make me feel emotionally and physically?
- Which movements connect me to my body?
- Which movements do I enjoy?

If you like to self-monitor, shifting your monitoring to the things you want to grow more of can have a powerful effect. For example, you could fill in a chart like this below in your notebook. Write down some of the forms of exercise you do, and things that you want to grow.

Type of movement	Date	Connection to body (0–10)	Improved stress? (0–10)	Improved mood? (0–10)
yoga	11/7	8	10	9
treadmill	11/9	2	7	3
West African dance	11/12	7	10	10

Practice mindful movement. Mindfulness is paying attention to the present moment, without judgment. Bring your full attention to what you are feeling, seeing, and sensing as you move, and let go of critical thoughts as you do so. Choose activities that support you in listening to your body from the inside out. Yoga, NIA, dance classes, and movement in nature are all great ways to increase what we call *embodiment*, which is your awareness of your physical sensations, movements, and emotional states. While moving your body, pay attention to what it feels like on the inside and how it connects you to what is happening on the outside.

Find movement mentors. I (Diana) found my first movement mentor at a yoga class for beginners taught by Wanda Be. Wanda showed me that movement didn't have to be painful but could be playful, gentle, and loving. In my thirties I started following Katy's work, and learned that movement could also be integrated into my daily life, doing chores with my kids, walking with my clients, and growing some of my own food. Who are your movement mentors? Write their names and where you can get inspired by them in your notebook. Spend more time (online, in print, or in person) with people who inspire values-aligned movement, and stop spending time on people and platforms who send unhealthy or rigid messages about movement.

Rethinking Movement
Making Friends with Movement

Problematic relationships with movement have this in common: There is not much enjoyment gained from the physical activity itself. Instead, exercise is used to offer a release from stress, unease, or dissatisfaction, or to improve self-esteem. Discovering the types of physical activity you enjoy and that enrich your life in multiple ways is a good benchmark to keep in mind as you develop a new motivation and get back to nourishing yourself with movement.

When it comes to moving more, get social. Meet your friends for coffee and a hike, or instead of driving to a fancy dinner, meet at someone's house for a cocktail then walk to the restaurant. Take a movement class you've always been curious about and ask some pals to join you. Play hoops or kick the soccer ball in your front yard and ask the neighbors to come over. Run a local 5k. Volunteer as a dog walker at the local animal rescue. Build a big flower garden. Take a frisbee to the park.

You're not alone. Exercise has long been framed as an atonement tool, and feeling punished by movement—moving despite injuries, forsaking others or other fun, feeling like it's in control of you—can feel like just par for the course. But physical activity is more like the axis of human culture: a tool for labor, for transportation, and for celebration. To help stay in a healthy relationship with exercise, find the types of movement that allow you to connect with and celebrate yourself and others every day.

2

I Don't Have Enough Time!

Every day, we each spend twenty-four hours over five domains: sleep, leisure, occupation, transportation, and home. There are so many "to dos" in each of these categories, and four out of five adults report that they have too much to do and not enough time to do it. We want to move our bodies more, but exercise is forced to compete with other important priorities like parenting, work, and sleep, especially if you are a working parent or in a family with limited resources. Does this sound familiar?

In this section, we'll be exploring how you can change your relationship with time. I (Diana) will be offering new tools when it comes to time, especially when it seems like our values might be in conflict with each other.

While time is measurable in terms of hours and minutes and is seemingly fixed, our perception of time, including the time we have available, is somewhat malleable. For example, when you are more fully present in a moment, you are likely to feel like you have more time available, experience less time pressure, and feel greater satisfaction with how you use your time.

And I (Katy) am going to show you how to increase the amount of time you have available in each day through something I call "stacking your life." Every day we complete a long list of tasks, each task usually fulfilling one need at a time. Stacking your life involves looking for tasks, or ways of doing tasks, that meet more than one need at a time. In this way, you can use just one period of time to take care of multiple needs at once, opening up more time in your day. Because movement and human bodies go all the way back to the beginning, movement layers quite well into all the domains of our life. Movement doesn't need to compete with our other needs; it can actually become a conduit for taking care of all the other things we humans must do daily.

Skipping movement when we feel time-crunched might seem to free up time, but it doesn't, really. Biologically our bodies need the movement, so when they don't get it on the regular, we accumulate an ever-growing deficit that can create disease or injury, which eventually forces us to slow down and take the time. And even the way we feel about time is affected by us choosing to move. When research participants spent their time exercising, they ended up feeling like they had *more* spare time, not less. In fact, UCLA professor Dr. Cassie Holmes, author of *The Happier Hour*, gives her students the assignment to move their body thirty minutes a day, in order to increase their feeling of "time affluence."

Creating a sustainable approach to prioritizing movement in our busy schedules isn't about squeezing in yet another activity. Instead, it's about getting present in the time we have and aligning our actions with what truly matters to us. A lack of time might not even be the deeper issue at hand! If you've been feeling strapped for time, slow down, and spend some time in this chapter. It's about time!

Reason 8: I don't have enough time to exercise; I have too much other work to do, and too many family responsibilities.

You sound like you have a full plate, with work and family taking up a lot of your time. When we're juggling home and work responsibilities, our mind might tell us that there's just no time to move. As a result, our days can feel like we're rushing from one thing to the next, doing more and more but never enough. It feels like we're rushing through life, rather than being in it—or in our bodies, for that matter.

The human mind is a master at categorizing and labeling things. Categorizing helps us make sense of the world, but it can also restrict our thinking. For example, what do you think counts as exercise? If you think movement is something that has to happen in a certain location or context, then you might not notice all the ways you could fit movement in alongside your other need-to-dos. If squatting is something that has to happen in a gym, for example, you may not notice the many squats you could do outside of the gym—like when you're picking up toys, grabbing pots from your lower kitchen cabinets, or digging in the garden. But squats in these contexts are also valuable, and they might be easier to fit in.

Your mind might also be categorizing time as being for work *or* family *or* exercise, which makes it harder to see the many ways these categories can overlap. Keeping these categorized as separate may be eating up your time. It takes time to transition between them, and you miss out on how they can benefit and enhance each other. For instance, if you go on a walk with your partner and talk out a problem you're having at work, is that family time? Work time? Exercise time? Or all three? When you step out of your mind's rigid categories, you free yourself to move in many domains at once—to stack your life!

Either/Or Thinking

Getting more flexible with how you look at movement and time can open up space in your day. Either/or thinking is when you see only one possibility as true—you don't see the in-between, or rainbow of options, because you are stuck in black-and-white, dichotomous ways of viewing the world. You might be thinking of movement as an either/or activity. *Either I am taking care of my family or I am moving my body. Either I am working or I am exercising.* The fact is, there are a lot of creative ways you can move your body while also tending to the different domains of your life. Let's use cognitive flexibility—unsticking ourselves from our thoughts by seeing them as simply thoughts, not truths—to become aware of our thinking patterns so that we can find them more easily.

Are you caught in either/or thinking when it comes to time and movement? Consider some common either/or mind blocks:

- Either I am with my kids or I am exercising.
- Either I am getting work done or I am getting my walk in.
- Either I am outside with my family or I am taking care of dinner.
- Either I am doing housework or I am doing my stretches.

You are getting cognitively flexible, or unhooking from your thoughts, every time you step back and look at them like this. You're like a fish being released from a hook: You don't have to get tugged around by your thoughts. Notice your mind's tendency to be absolute when it comes to how much time you think you have to move.

What are some of your either/or thinking blocks? How does your mind's habit of categorizing constrain your movement?

Go ahead and jot down in your notebook a few either/or thoughts that impact how much time you think you have to move. Just noticing these thoughts is an intervention in itself! Remember, with cognitive flexibility you can have a thought, but you don't have to believe it to be true.

Both/And Thinking

Our mind wants to live in the land of "either/or," but the reality is that multiple things can be true at the same time. Most things exist more in the middle world of "both/and." Both/and thinking is when you realize many possibilities can be happening at the same time—you can see the in-between and the rainbow of options, because you have flexible ways of viewing the world.

When you feel strapped for time, you can shift your thinking to both/and statements to discover a little wiggle room. Try finishing these both/and thinking statements below. Get creative. Is there a way you can both move and engage with the important domains of your life? Go back to your notebook and see if you can change some of your either/or statements to both/and.

- I can *both* be with my kids *and* move my body by…
- One way I can *both* work *and* walk is…
- I can *both* be outside with my family *and* take care of dinner if I…
- I can *both* do housework *and* get some stretching by…

Pick a both/and thought to try this week. Open up your either/or mind, and let the categories blur a little around the edges. Notice how your relationship with time changes when you have a more flexible mindset.

Rethinking Movement
Both/And-ing Common Either/Ors

There are many times when we are cognitively flexible—we are ready and willing to both/and—but we can't figure out creative solutions ourselves. When everyone around us is stuck in the "not enough time" paradigm, we never see a model of stacking movement. So let's explore creative, stack-your-life solutions to the barriers above to help get your creative juices flowing.

Either I am with my kids or I am exercising. You might flip your thinking here: Kids are practically live-in personal trainers if you let them be. All that lifting, bending, carrying, and following around babies and toddlers will keep your arm, leg, and core muscles moving a lot more than before you had them. Little ones love moving around outside, so if you're feeling too still with your little ones, add a daily walk or trip to the park and you can all get the movement you need. Getting everyone out for movement is part of caretaking—kids need lots of outside movement too, and this one activity (everyone going outside) meets multiple needs at once.

Doing some or all of a walk to and from school with school-age kids can turn this chore into not only movement for you and your kids, but a chance for them to blow off some of their sedentary steam or debrief their day with you. Or if homework keeps everyone sitting down inside, suggest going outside and quiz spelling words, math facts, and poetry memorization on the move.

Either I am getting work done or I am getting my walk in. Which elements of your work can be more dynamic? Can some phone calls be taken while you're on foot? When your coworkers need to meet, suggest a walking meeting. Instead of sending emails to the coworker a short walk away, get in more steps by going to see them in person throughout the day. Use your work breaks and lunchtime to log some time walking up and down in-office stairs or head outside for a nearby powerwalk. Find the minutes!

Either I am outside with my family or I can take care of dinner. I (Katy) really disliked having to go inside to start working on dinner when my kids were little. Not only did I not want to give up the dose of nature for my own body, everyone tended to want to come inside with me, which made *everyone* stop playfully moving their bodies (and start getting grumpy!). Still, we needed to eat.

I began bringing some of my dinner prep tasks, like chopping veggies, outside. There wasn't usually any real reason to go inside to prepare food. Instead, I was able to be outside while my kids kept playing, work on dinner, and sit on the ground (using the "laundry stretches" on page 74), so I increased my movement too.

Other ways to stack mealtime with movement include cooking or eating your meals outside more often, or layering a meal with some family walking time: Pack simple dinners and take everyone out for an evening meal on foot.

Either I am doing housework or I am doing my stretches. A flexible mindset can actually help you with flexibility! Housework is an excellent place to fit in some of the exercise you're looking for, whether it's cardiovascular (shake out those rugs, push that lawn mower), big-body strength (stacking wood, carrying loads of laundry), or stretching—you just have to adjust the way you approach a task.

I (Katy) fit in a lot of my hip and leg stretching while folding laundry. There's always laundry (am I right?), which means there are also always opportunities to stretch. I put everything on the floor around me and start working in a straddle-stretch position (legs in a V), then move to sitting with crossed legs, then sitting with my legs folded beneath me to stretch my knees and ankles. I'm just doing one task, but by changing *the way* I do it—from sitting on the couch or standing at a table to getting down on the floor—I stack it with stretches, getting more done in the same period of time.

And I (Diana) get good carrying movement when I'm lugging in loads of groceries for two adolescent boys. Changing my mind to think this is both good for my family and a nutritious movement for me makes the task feel more bearable, plus I can skip the farmer's carry at the gym, which saves me time!

These are all examples of "stacks" that layer movement into what you were already doing, no extra time needed. What are ways you can fit this principle into your own life?

Reason 9: Once the kids are finally in bed and I have those few precious moments for myself, I prioritize my favorite hobbies (sewing, crafting, crocheting, reading), which do not involve that much movement.

Your time *is* precious, and it's wonderful that you are prioritizing enjoyable activities such as sewing and reading. You may gravitate to these hobbies because they are pleasurable, meaningful, and interesting. According to researchers Oishi and Westgate, these three components—pleasure (also called hedonia), meaning (also called eudemonia), and interest (also called psychological richness)—are what make up a well-lived life. What if movement could be considered another one of those precious moments for yourself, contributing to a life well lived?

Your Well-Lived Life

Make movement pleasurable. Have you lost the *joy* of movement? Dr. Kelly McGonigal writes in her book *The Joy of Movement*, "Movement is one of the most powerful ways to experience joy, because it both grounds us in the present moment and gives us a sense of freedom and possibility." When activities are pleasurable, we want to do them again. When you are tired, stressed, or feeling down, it helps to have a list of movements that you are drawn to because you love them.

Jot down a list of some movements that bring you joy. To help with this brainstorming exercise, consider:

- What type of movements did you love as a kid?
- What type of movements do you look forward to doing?
- Which movements feel good in your body?
- Which movements connect you to others?

- What types of movement sound fun, interesting, or pleasant?

- When was the last time you moved your body and enjoyed it?

Are there any movements that you could bring into the end of the day that would feel pleasurable in the way that reading, sewing, and other hobbies do?

The more you focus on enjoying movement, the more motivated you will be to keep moving.

Make movement meaningful. Moving your body more isn't always pleasurable. Sometimes it takes a bit of effort, discomfort, and inertia-busting to get going. Tapping into the bigger reasons you want to move your body can increase your motivation, even when it's difficult. In fact, being told all the reasons you should exercise can make you exercise less, but reflecting on the reasons movement is personally relevant to you is likely to increase your time spent moving.

Go back and explore your values (pages 15–19). Pause and reflect on why moving your body is personally relevant to you.

- Why is movement important to you?

- How will moving your body make a difference to your life in the long term?

- How does moving your body impact your health, your relationships, your work, your wellbeing?

- What are the three top reasons you want to move your body more?

Write some of these reasons down and put this list with your sewing and crafting materials. When you pick up your end-of-day craft, it will help remind you why you want to make time for movement too.

Make movement interesting. You are more likely to want to spend your free time moving if you find it interesting and engaging. We are naturally motivated to grow, learn new things, and develop competence. Movement can offer you a challenge, a shift in perspective, and novelty. Together, these qualities build what's called "psychological richness." Psychological richness refers to having a life filled with interesting and diverse experiences, which can contribute to your overall sense of enrichment, even if it doesn't directly increase happiness or life satisfaction. In fascinating studies on this topic, researchers found that students who studied abroad reported feeling more psychologically enriched compared to those who stayed on campus, though they didn't necessarily feel happier or find greater meaning in life. Similarly, participants in escape rooms—a game where you solve puzzles to "escape" a themed room—felt more psychologically rich as the rooms became more difficult, though their happiness levels didn't increase. Movement works the same way—when you take on new, interesting, and challenging physical activities, you can grow more psychologically rich!

You can up the psychological richness of physical activity by choosing activities that are challenging, novel, and slightly outside your comfort zone. Choose activities that spark feelings of curiosity and wonder (I wonder what it would be like to take an online dance class in the evening? Or take a walk through my neighborhood in the moonlight?)

Pull out your notebook and make a list of physical activities that interest you, offer a perspective shift, or stretch you in some way. Include activities you have never tried and activities that you already do and want to get more skilled at. What new, interesting, curious movement can you add to your precious evening time this week?

For a bonus, see if you find some ways of moving that fit all three of these qualities. Which movements are pleasurable, meaningful, *and* psychologically rich? Engaging in activities like this make your life well-lived, and worth spending your precious time on.

Rethinking Movement
Dynamic Up Your Hobbies

With the exception of reading, these activities you've listed are actually comprised of "making movements" that go way back with most of our ancestors. The activities you're drawn to sound restful, and might be appropriate for you in the evening, especially if the day has left you physically or attentionally fatigued. Assuming that's so, there are two ways we can work on balancing your movement diet. The first is to add movement to your favorite tasks. Reading, for example, pairs well with many stretches, like spinal twists, legs up the wall, and hip openers—no extra time needed. If you want more vigorous movement, reading (or listening to an audiobook) while riding a stationary bike can also be a good stack, and of course audiobooks can come on a walk with you. Train different muscles more by stretching your sewing patterns out on the living room floor. Floor sitting, whether it's while sewing or crocheting, gives joints and muscles different shapes to try, and that's all exercise is, really: getting into different shapes or intensities that cause your body to keep growing in strength and skill.

The second way to get more movement starts with questioning why you're saving all your movement for after the kids are in bed. You might have quite practical reasons, or maybe your entire daytime holds space for you to get the bigger-body movement you're wanting (some other answers in the book might help you with that), leaving your evenings free for the quiet making movements you find restful. And of course, you can always approach this issue in both ways—add movement to your evening "making time" while also weaving movement throughout your daytime.

Reason 10: If I don't have enough time to do my full workout, I won't do it. I think it doesn't count.

We all carry around rules, "shoulds," and beliefs about what counts as exercise. But when you hold an exercise rule tightly, it can really limit how, when, and how much you move. Many of our mind's rules are either outdated, unhelpful, or inaccurate. There can be so many influences on the way we think! For instance, you might have adopted certain "exercise rules" from sources like podcasts, physical education teachers, coaches, or, if you are me (Diana), Jane Fonda VHS workout tapes from the 1990s. I can still hear her saying we needed to "feel the burn" to know it was working. And you may be adhering to these rules without asking yourself, "Is this rule helpful given my movement goals?" It sounds like you have a rule that you need spend a magic number of consecutive minutes for movement to count. This is a pretty common belief, even though research shows that short bouts of moderate-intensity physical activity (known as exercise snacking) are associated with similar reductions in cardiovascular risk factors to longer, continuous sessions, as well as the health benefits of staying lightly active throughout the day

When you notice a rule is getting in the way of you choosing to move, it's a good time to practice **cognitive flexibility**. Step back from the rule your mind is telling you, and recognize that although it may feel true, it doesn't have to direct your behavior. When you say, "If I can't do my full workout, then I won't do it," how long is a full workout in your mind? Is it about time? About a certain set of moves to be done in a day? Do they have to all be done at once? What are your rules about what constitutes a "full workout"? And what are other rules around movement you might have? This may be just one of many movement rules that might be interfering with you getting the movement you want.

Let's explore this further. In your notebook, label a page *My Exercise Rules* and jot your rules down. Are any of these familiar?

- It has to be at least thirty minutes to count.
- I need to do it at the gym.
- I have to do ten reps.
- I must walk ten thousand steps.
- I should stay for the whole exercise class.
- I should be wearing exercise gear, so I have to do it later.

A lot of these thoughts start with *I have to, I need to, I must,* or *I should.* Phrases like these are often clues you are stuck in an inflexible rule. They are also limiting, because what if you only have twenty-five minutes—does that mean you don't go for a walk? Or, you really enjoy swimming and you hop in the pool for a few quick laps—does that not count? If you only have an hour at lunch, could you leave yoga class a little early, or do you have rules you've made up about having to stay for the whole time for it to count? Do you not allow yourself to do just part of a class, video, or routine? Or maybe you don't bother to check if it's actually an external rule, instead of one you made up?

Class rules

I (Katy) tell my students, in person and in my studio's newsletter, that if there's some conflict with the way class time lines up with their other obligations, coming in late or leaving early are fine, and I note how they can do this without disrupting the experience for me as the teacher, or for the other students. Many exercise teachers are out there trying to help folks move, so I encourage you to reach out to your movement class instructor and ask about the possibility of attending shorter portions of offerings. So many times we assume the rules in our head match up with the rules of others, but communication is the best way to see what's actually going on. I (Diana) have attended yoga studios that make it very clear not to enter at the beginning of class during meditation or leave during the quiet resting time at the end of class. So, if I need to leave early, I let the instructor know and make sure I am out of there as they are winding down. This allows me to fit in a class midday between clients, and be a better therapist when I return because of it! There will always be more and less flexible people and institutions, but you'll never know until you ask!

To get more flexible with your rules, it helps to consider whether they support or derail you from your values and goals. Go through your list of rules and ask yourself, "How helpful is this rule? Are there times when I want to hold it more lightly? Are there times when it supports my values and goals?" Then get even more flexible with your rules by breaking some on purpose.

Break Some of Your Exercise Rules

Just because your mind has rules about doing exercise "right" doesn't mean you have to follow them. When you break a rule on purpose, you strengthen your ability to act independently from your mind's inflexible thoughts and rules. This builds autonomy and confidence that you, not your thoughts, are in charge of your movement plans. It also is kind of fun to be a movement rebel! When I (Diana) lead a webinar or training, I love to break the rule that many participants might have about needing to be seated to participate. I encourage them to grab their phone and take a walk as they listen, or to lie on the floor or move about their space.

Start by breaking your rule about needing to do a full workout. On purpose, take committed action and do half, three quarters, or even only 10 percent of your workout. You can leave it at that, or add more time to move later in the day. But be careful: Your mind will want to find a way to follow the rule (e.g., so that it all adds up to a "real" workout). Every time this happens, unstick yourself from the thought that it has to be a full workout to count and recommit to breaking the rule again. Remember that every time you break your mind's rules, you create a more flexible mind, and chances are you will end up moving more, not less!

Next, pick a few of the other rules you listed in your notebook and commit to breaking them on purpose. If you have a rule that you have to do ten reps, try doing twenty or just three. If you have a rule that you have to exercise at a certain intensity for it to count, walk instead of run, or go to a level 1 class instead of a level 2. Be playful with it and show your mind who's in charge here. Don't let your rules boss you around! Prove to yourself that you, not your rules, get to decide how you will move.

Rethinking Movement
Movement "Snacks" Are Also Nourishing

While the idea of a "training session" (a dedicated bout of movement outside of other daily activities for improving fitness for athletic or military performance) has been around since early civilizations, the widespread concept of "workouts" as we think of them today have only been around since the 1960s. The idea of workouts as popularized by Dr. Ken Cooper (father of aerobic fitness science), Jane Fonda, and the Weider brothers (bodybuilders) came about at a time when many people were transitioning from more active to less active lifestyles. The positive effects of a workout (and there are many) have perhaps created the belief that a workout is the only way we can nourish our bodies with movement, but really, doing different movements throughout the day has adequately nourished the human body for a million years.

That all being said, many societies are now much more sedentary than before, and movement isn't part of many people's daily activities like it was in our grandparents' day—which is why exercise has become a helpful concept for many. Ironically, we've got a new problem: It seems there's no time to fit in a full workout, which is why time seems like such a big barrier to movement.

Kinesiology, the study of human movement, really started off as the study of exercise, but it has since expanded beyond the narrower concepts of athletics and workouts. Now there's more and more research and promotion of "movement snacking" instead of being still most of the day and then trying to find the time to get in a "full workout." Looking for multiple places to fit a few minutes here or there to get in a burst of activity is an excellent alternative to a workout (maybe even better, if it means you are able to fit the movement in).

Another way to break this limiting movement rule could be to list all the movements that go into your full workout, and pepper them throughout the day. Get twenty minutes of lung-challenging movements first thing, do your lunge series and stretches on your lunch break, and save push-ups and sit-ups for the evening while you're watching your favorite show.

There's no denying that getting a long workout is great for improving endurance, and it often feels good just to have an extended break from all the other stuff you need to do. That being said, any movement we fit in "counts" as far as our physiology is concerned.

Reason 11: I love walking in the mornings, but I feel guilty not spending that time with my husband before he goes to work. If I wait till he's gone, then I'm not there when our seventeen-year-old gets up, and I feel guilty she's waking up to an empty house. This is self-assigned guilt; no one else cares.

It's hard when you feel like you're being pulled in many directions at once. Parental guilt is a common experience because we care so much! But guilt is a tricky emotion, because sometimes our guilt doesn't match the situation or is unjustified (e.g., parents often feel guilty for self-care, when it ultimately serves the whole family), or it demotivates us to pursue our goals and values. Like all emotions, guilt is neither good nor bad, and can be helpful in some contexts. Humans likely evolved guilt as a mechanism to promote our social connections, and guilt is a useful emotion when it motivates us to course-correct behavior that violates our own values or moral code. Guilt is good if it motivates you to apologize when you have harmed someone, or do that thing you know you are avoiding. But in your case it sounds like your guilt is not supported by the facts of the situation ("this is self-assigned guilt; no one else cares"), and it's getting in the way of spending time doing what nourishes you ("I love walking in the mornings!").

When you are consumed by guilt, you are likely to act in ways that get rid of your bad feeling (see "motivation" types, pages 13–14), rather than making the choices that are best for you and your family.

So how can you address your feelings of time guilt and still get out and walk?

Connect to your values. When you describe feeling guilty for not spending time with your husband or being there for your daughter, what

I (Diana) also hear is that you value being present with your family and taking care of your needs. Rather than getting entangled in guilt, ask yourself, what is important to me here? How can I be present for my family and for myself? Maybe it's leaving a little note for your daughter to call you when she wakes up so you can walk and say good morning. Or, it's getting up a little earlier so you can walk first and then spend time with your husband (do you need to be home as soon as he wakes up, or will he spend some time in the shower and getting dressed when you wouldn't be talking to him anyway? Can you time your return so you can drink your coffee together?). What would it look like to live out both of these values of being present for your family and taking care of your needs in a more flexible way? Remember that there are hundreds of ways to express your values—you're only bound by your creativity!

Take opposite action. You said, "This is self-assigned guilt. No one else cares." There's a technique I often use in therapy called "opposite action" that's particularly helpful when our emotions are derailing us from acting effectively. Opposite action involves doing the opposite of what the emotion tells you to do. Opposite action helps you break up your emotion's hold over you by demonstrating that you can have an emotion without it ruling your behavior. Opposite action is a form of committed action, and you can do it in these steps:

1. Notice when guilt shows up for you.

2. Is your guilt helpful in supporting your values and goals? If yes, listen to your guilt and adjust your behavior. If not, continue with the next steps.

3. Notice the urge to avoid feeling guilty. What does it urge you to do? Is it to stay home? Skip your walk? Override your physical and psychological needs? Apologize for having needs?

4. Act the opposite: Make it known to your family that you are choosing to go for a walk because it's great for you. Don't apologize. You can even show opposite action with your body by changing your body posture from guilty to

confident. Stand tall, keep your voice steady and clear, and walk with gusto.

5. Remind yourself that you can feel guilty, but you don't have to *act* guilty, and/or change your behavior accordingly.

6. Open up to and accept the discomfort that comes with this! The more you take action that's opposite to your emotion, the easier it will get.

Try both/and thinking. Pay attention to your thinking here and make your either/or thoughts flexible. It seems like you think walking and family care are mutually exclusive choices—that you have to choose between time with your family and time walking. But really, walking and family care may positively influence each other. For example, on days you walk, how does it impact your mood, attention, and engagement with your family? You might notice you are more patient with your teenager, more empathetic when your husband talks about his day ahead, or more cheery and enjoyable to be around. Your walking might enhance the quality of the time you spend with your family, and when you spend quality time with your family, you might feel freer and less guilty about walking! Try turning a few either/or statements about walking and family care into both/and statements.

Rethinking Movement
Moving Together

In addition to your morning walk, during which you might prefer to be on your own, you can also connect with your husband and teen by inviting them to walk at different times too.

Or, an early, before-work walk with your husband might be a great way to spend time together, get some of your daily planning done, and get you both a dose of walking, nature, and morning sun.

You can also ask if there are physical activities they want to do any time of day that you can join in. You'll end up with quality time, movement needs met, and learning something new yourself.

Reason 12: I work ten to twelve hours a day just to eke out a living. I'm also sandwich generation, caretaking an elderly parent and grandkids. Not much time or energy left for exercise.

When daily life is demanding, with limited income, long working hours, and the added responsibility of supporting an elderly parent and grandchildren, it can feel impossible to find the time and energy to exercise. You aren't alone. There is a correlation between family income and the percentage of adults who meet the guidelines for aerobic and muscle-strengthening activities. A 2020 study found that only 10 percent of women and 16 percent of men with family income below the Federal Poverty Level (FDL) met physical activities guidelines. The percentage of those meeting activity guidelines was doubled for those with high incomes. Research also shows that caregivers report difficulty meeting exercise guidelines for a wide range of reasons, including limitations in daily activity options, lack of time, and limited social support for maintaining an exercise routine.

It's especially crucial for you to get physical activity given your responsibilities and stressors. At the same time, it's especially hard for you to do it, given the loads you carry. How to move forward?

Cultivate Inner Resources

Financial strain and caretaking can create stress that's hard on the body. Even when life doesn't offer much relief, there are psychological tools that can help you manage stress more effectively. For instance, research at UCSF by Dr. Alexandra Crosswell reveals that caregivers who find meaning in their work, fully accept their experiences, and maintain a sense of anticipation or something to look forward to show healthier physiological responses to stress. These caregivers not only cope better emotionally but also exhibit improved metabolic and cellular health, including lower inflammation and better maintenance of telomeres—the protective caps at the ends of our chromosomes that keep us from aging too quickly.

Here's how you could apply these protective mindsets, even with limited time and external resources.

Find purpose. Caregivers who have a deeper sense of purpose in their caregiving tend to cope better with stress. Try infusing some purpose into your physical activity. Maybe it's motivating for you to be an example for your grandkids when you model physical activity. Or, you want to use this as a chance to encourage your parent to be active with you. What message do you want to convey about maintaining an active lifestyle throughout life? Demonstrate the values you want to instill in your grandkids and your parent about movement when you are with them.

Practice acceptance. Rejecting reality, or wishing things to be different from how they are, makes our stress feel even more unbearable. When you feel stressed or overwhelmed with a long day of work or caregiving, remember that all you have to handle is just this moment. Practicing acceptance with physical activity may include accepting that your movement might look different during this phase of your life. Pushing strollers, walking slowly with your parents, and carrying groceries are all ways you can move and care for your loved ones at the same time. Instead of going to a gym or doing a bout of vigorous movement, you might need to adjust to easier movements that you find restful while still taking care of your body's needs.

Generate joyful movement. Research suggests that shifting your mind to joy can be an antidote to stress. In the morning, think about your day ahead and ways to incorporate movement that you look forward to. This is something you can list in your notebook every morning. You can put at the top of the page *Joyful Movement Plan* and list three things that stack physical activity with caregiving that you look forward to. Perhaps you love tossing a ball, exploring the outdoors, digging in the sandbox, pushing grandkids on the swings, or playing on the floor together. Make sure to include ways to engage your parents in pleasurable movement. Could you plan a leisurely stroll outdoors or take them with you to the community center or park? Can you ask for their guidance in your garden or with another outdoor chore, where they can tell you what to do based on their many years of experience, and you can do the moves involved, with as much physical help as they're able to give? Is there a way to move with your parent and grandkids at the same time? I (Katy) have many memories of gathering walnuts from beneath a tree when I was very little. We then spent afternoons shelling them with the community elders in the backyard. Everyone was active and contributing, and it was joyful for all of us.

Make it a point to experience the joy of sharing moments of movement with your family every day, and savor the time you have with them.

Cultivate External Resources: Vitamin Community

When we struggle financially, meeting the demands of more immediate, short-term needs takes up our mental energy and tangible resources. This is something that health researchers are recognizing more and more: Exercise isn't only a matter of motivation.

Caretaking moves

Caretaking can involve quite a bit of movement, and many jobs are physical, too. Are you counting those movements towards your daily physical activity? In a study of hotel room cleaners (a job that involves walking many steps, lifting and carrying heavy things, bending, twisting, and picking up objects from the floor), 67 percent reported not exercising regularly, despite most meeting the Surgeon General's recommendations for an active lifestyle most days. Researchers then created two groups of workers. One group was educated on how movement done during their workday was "good exercise," and the other group wasn't told or taught anything. Four weeks later, the first group, who understood that their workday movement counted, perceived themselves as getting more exercise than before (even though the amount they moved did not change), and, incredibly, they also showed physiological benefits associated with getting more movement: decreases in weight, blood pressure, body fat, waist-to-hip ratio, and body mass index. The researchers concluded that when the hotel workers believed they were exercising, their body responded as if they were, similarly to how your body responds to a placebo medication.

This could be the case, and it's also possible that when we realize the work we are doing is beneficial in some additional ways, we might begin doing it with more vigor or with a better attitude. Maybe the simple realization that we're getting the movement we need is enough to decrease stress and its negative impacts!

In any case, we'll keep beating this drum: Movement shows up in many beneficial forms that aren't exercise. And mind-set matters when it comes to movement. What are you already doing that you aren't counting?

Rethinking Movement
Caretaking Movements

As a culture we're starting to recognize how emotionally taxing caretaking is, and I'd add that it's also incredibly *physically* taxing. Lifting and moving the person you're caring for, doing the bulk of all housework and errands, and running on diminished sleep are all things that demand a lot from your body. Caretakers can be exhausted and find themselves sore a lot of the time.

I (Katy) spent a short period of time caring for an ailing parent, and because I'm always trying to move as well as figure out where movement can fit into everyday life, I played with stacking movement into my caretaking work. For example, when it came to laundry, I found benefit in the movement of putting it up and taking it down off a rack or line, and would fold it on the floor so I could stretch my hips at the same time. I did small stretches in the kitchen (stretching my calves at the sink!) and while loading the dishwasher and washing machine.

I also found that while longer walks were not possible, I could take five-minute walks, multiple times throughout the day, even if they were just a quick jaunt around the outside of the house. If I had coverage to do an errand, I would opt to do it on foot.

Tending to yourself physically in a way that doesn't require extra time and money might help address some of *your* many needs if you spend a lot of time tending to someone else's needs. When you stack your movement with your caretaking work, you'll be able to do your tasks with much less injury, and you'll be taking better care of yourself as you do your important work.

Note that everything above does not mean you couldn't still benefit from a long bout of movement or a long time away from caretaking. Everybody needs a break sometimes! But we can also reframe the idea that caretaking only benefits the one being taken care of. Many families deal with years of caretaking, and what can help you through is to see that often the needs of more than one person can be met in a caretaking scenario. This can even be true physically. And if an hour away from caretaking is not possible for you—or it is, but you'd rather not spend it exercising—you have options.

Reason 13: I feel that it's selfish to do something for my own body and soul when other people need something from me.

Why is this question in the TIME chapter? Because often when we think of taking care of ourselves as selfish behavior, we are ultimately saying, "I am using my time for them or me." When we think we have to split our time in this way, we have a misconception that doing something for ourselves is somehow separate from doing something that is also good for others. There's that "either/or" thinking again! In reality, caring for your body and soul can be an act of self-compassion that allows you to better show up for the people who need you.

Nurturing your body through physical activity is one of the kindest things you can do for yourself, and it also spills over to those you love. It's very "both/and!"

So how do you know if your physical activity is an act of self-compassion, or if you're just being selfish? Let's take a look at self-compassion and selfishness more closely. While the "self" might be a shared feature of self-compassion and selfishness, they are quite different. Self-compassion is treating yourself with the same kindness you would offer a good friend, especially when you are having a hard time. Selfishness is prioritizing your own needs at the expense of others. Look at these lists and notice the differences between the two.

SELF-COMPASSION	SELFISHNESS
Being kind, understanding, and supportive towards yourself, especially during struggle	Being primarily concerned with personal gain and pleasure, often at the expense of others
Balancing your wellbeing with an awareness of communal welfare	Focusing solely on your own needs and desires without regard for others
Improving relationships by building empathy, connection, and mutual support	Harming relationships by isolating, disconnecting, and neglecting others' needs
Relating to others, feeling not better or less than others, interconnected	Feeling better than others, separate, and individualistic

Physical activity can be done selfishly or self-compassionately, depending on its impact on others. Here are some examples. Where can you fit in taking time to give your body the movement it needs?

SELF-COMPASSIONATE PHYSICAL ACTIVITY	SELFISH PHYSICAL ACTIVITY
Using physical activity as a way to improve how you show up in other responsibilities	Using physical activity to avoid other responsibilities
Getting active to reduce stress, improve mood, protect mental health	Being physically active in a way that causes stress to your family, workplace, or friends

Incorporating physical activity into your daily activities to make them more enriching and beneficial for your wellbeing	Ignoring others' needs so you can be physically active
Using physical activity to care for your physical health, chronic pain, illness prevention	Using physical activity in a way that causes others to be unwell or in pain (e.g., working out at the gym when you are sick and spreading germs)

As you can see, when physical activity becomes about meeting only your needs, harms relationships, and makes you feel "better than" others, it can be selfish. For example, if you cancel plans or regularly show up late to picking up your friends because you wanted to hit the gym instead, or you always choose exercise over spending time with your family, it may be crossing the line to selfishness. But there are likely way more times when physical activity is an act of self-compassion that ultimately *benefits* those around you. If staying active can help you be a more patient friend or less irritable partner, your people will thank you! And when you acknowledge that everyone, including you, deserves and needs the time to move their body, it's an act of self-compassion. Can you add to this list? When is taking time for your physical activity an act of self-compassion, and does it ever become selfish? Get out your notebook and make two columns, one for self-compassion and one for selfishness. Add your own examples.

The idea here is to find the sweet spot where your physical activity is beneficial for your wellbeing and also benefits others. When it supports your inner and outer harmony. You may find that by taking care of your body, you have more energy and resources to be there for others when they need you. With self-compassion, you recognize our interdependence: *When you take care of you, and I take care of me, we can take better care of each other.*

It's not always easy straight away, but fortunately self-compassion is a skill that you can develop with practice. At first it may feel awkward or different to do something good for your body and soul, but just because it feels different doesn't make it wrong. Below are some self-compassion practices you can try on a regular basis. They will get easier over time.

Embody a Compassionate Self

How you hold your body impacts how you feel and think (a concept that psychologists call *embodied cognition*). For example, adopting an upright, open posture can lead to feelings of confidence, whereas slumping or closing off your body can contribute to feelings of sadness or defeat. This is because the way we carry our bodies can send feedback to the brain that shapes our emotional state. Embodying a compassionate self involves stepping into a version of you that is strong, wise, and caring, and wants the best for you. When you take on a compassionate posture, facial expression, and even tone of voice, it has been shown to help you feel more safe and relaxed and have more compassion for others. Try the embodiment visualization below next time you engage in a physical activity.

1. Take a few long breaths. Bring to mind someone you admire for being courageous and strong. Imagine their brave heart is beating inside your body right now.

2. Next imagine someone you admire for being wise. Pretend that you can look through their eyes right now and see the world from this wise perspective.

3. Next imagine someone you admire for being balanced. Imagine you could breathe the way they breathe—slow, balanced, and at ease.

4. Finally, imagine someone you experience as kind, friendly, balanced, and warm. Take on their facial expression, their tone of voice, and their open posture.

5. Embody this compassionate version of you who is brave, wise, balanced, and kind. This is what it feels like to be

your compassionate self. How does this compassionate self think about caring for yourself with movement? What would they tell you?

6. Take a moment to write a compassionate statement down in your notebook. Write a statement that would be a helpful reminder when you feel like prioritizing movement is selfish. Here's an example:

   My Compassionate Self:

   Brave Heart (my sister Kathleen)

   Wise Eyes (Zen monk Thich Nhat Hanh)

   Balanced Breath (my friend Liz)

   Kind Face (my neighbor Cassie)

   My Compassionate Statement: When you take a brisk walk before you go help out your parents, you can better be there for them with your whole heart and attention.

7. Next time you feel selfish for taking care of your body, take on this physical posture, these eyes, this breath, this kind facial expression, and say your compassionate statement (aloud or in your mind!).

Enter the Flow of Compassion

Now that you have embodied compassion, you can allow it to flow three ways: giving compassion to yourself, giving compassion to others, and receiving compassion from others. Turn your physical activity into a flow of compassion so that you are giving as much as you receive.

Self-compassion. Physical activity can be a way to care for yourself when you're feeling low, stressed, or anxious. What physical activities best uplift your mood and enhance your overall wellbeing? Are there certain types of physical activity that work best for different emotions? For example, when I (Diana) am sad, I like to take a slow walk along the beach. There's something about the big blue space that gives room for grief. But when I am angry, I like to hike the hills behind my house. The steeper the better. And when I am stressed, there's nothing that can match a dunk in the cold ocean. When you tend to your emotions through movement in this way, it is a powerful act of self-compassion—you are acknowledging that you hurt and you are doing something about it.

Give compassion. You can also use physical activity to show support to others who are having a difficult time. For example, my (Diana's) family loves to join in on beach cleanups, trail building, and compost building to support the environment. When I have a client struggling with depression, I often give them the homework to go for a walk and ask a friend about their friend's problems, rather than ruminating on their own. Offer to take your neighbor's dog for a walk, to shovel their snow or drag their trashcans back in. It feels good to use your body to help others! Or you can extend compassion beyond your inner circle with movement by raising money for a cause you care about, such as organizing or joining in on a fundraising ride, swim, or walk.

Receive compassion. The final flow of compassion is taking in support from others. We all could use some support in staying active. And when you ask for help, you are also encouraging others to get active with you. For example, ask a friend to drive with you to exercise class, seek accountability from an online group, ask your partner to wake you up when they rise early for morning movement, or request movement-related gifts for special occasions, such as punch passes, workout attire, or active vacations. Let yourself receive the gift of compassion as you give it to others. That is how it flows! To you, from you, and within you.

When you feel like it's selfish to move your body, remember that movement can be an act of compassion. It not only benefits you, but it contributes positively to your relationships and the community at large. That is a good use of your time!

Rethinking Movement
Selfish and Lazy

We've already discussed why movements that are meaningful to you are so much easier to prioritize: they're value-driven! If you value being of service, look for ways of moving that stack with being supportive of others. If you're climate-conscious, choose active (human-powered) transportation when you can. If you're tending the needs of children—parenting, alloparenting (taking care of other people's kids), teaching, or social work—a stretching, yoga, or bodybuilding session that allows you to rest your mind and restore your body so you can *come back tomorrow and do it again* is part of your service package. It's good for you and ultimately good for others.

This isn't to say that all your movement needs to be in support of others. I (Katy) have this way of labeling myself lazy when I'm not being productive. I feel an urgency when it comes to "doing" and I'm motivated to "do" because I don't like the feeling of taking even a little bit of much-needed rest. Even when I'm sick, I'll catch myself thinking (or straight up saying aloud), *I'm so lazy*. While "lazy" is the label I give myself, at this point in my life I know I've just confused being lazy with not being productive right now. Is it possible to be lazy? Sure. But does taking a weekend nap, skipping a workout when I'm sore, or reading in bed all day when I'm sick mean I'm lazy? No. This is just nourishing myself with rest, and resting ultimately supports my ability to be productive. I bet it's something similar for you. You've got "selfish" confused with "not helping others right now." Now, you *might* be selfish (check those charts!), but we'd bet you're not being a jerk; you just feel motivated to avoid the feeling of the "not helping others right in this moment" label. Take a look around. Are you regularly serving others? Then go take that run, that class, OR THAT NAP. It's all good.

Reason 14: I'm burned out. I focus most of my energy on parenting two young kids and I have nothing left to give to exercise.

Every parent experiences stress. However, when stress becomes chronic to the point where you are exhausted, overwhelmed, and detached from your children, you are in what's called *parental burnout*. I (Diana) remember when my second son was born, being so burned out that some afternoons all I could do was lie on the ground and have my children crawl around me. I physically *could not* get up and do all the things I expected of myself. And I (Katy) am working on managing parental stress now that I'm parenting adolescents. There is no "easy age" when it comes to kids!

Parenting requires us to shift our perspective, and adjust our expectations and routines to match the changes that come with parenting. When you have too many demands on you and not enough internal or external resources to meet those demands, or if you can't adjust your expectations, you may burn out. Here are the three features of parental burnout. See which of these fit for you:

- Physical exhaustion: You feel emotionally drained by your role as a parent; you've reached the end of your tether.
- A sense of detachment: You distance yourself from your kids; you do the bare minimum.
- Ineffectiveness: You feel like you can't handle problems effectively or calmly. You are irritable, anxious, and having difficulty regulating your emotions.

To address your burnout and get you moving again, try some of the following tips.

Tips for Parental Exhaustion

Parenting is exhausting. In addition to the emotional and physical demands of parenting, many parents' sleep is disrupted by kids waking up or because they choose to have a few hours alone over a few more hours of sleep. This can wear you down over time. Turn exhaustion around by finding ways to insert more constructive and movement-based rest into your day. Get flexible in the way you think about rest. This takes a perspective shift. Rest doesn't only happen in a bed or on a couch. For example, getting the kids outside and into nature can help recalibrate your nervous system and reduce stress. Or get on the floor with them. It can feel restorative to lie on your belly and play a game of Uno, put your legs up the wall and read to them, or if you need a massage, let them walk on your back! The floor can feel grounding, and being down there is also a great way to connect with your kids, at their level. This way you'll be moving more parts, playing with your kids, and getting some rest.

Finally, make sure to mentally give yourself an end to the day. As a parent, your task list will never truly be complete. Your kids are probably making messes, dirtying laundry, and working up an appetite even as you read this. Regardless of how many items remain on your to-do list, establish a designated time to call it a day and step away. Accept the feelings of not getting it all done, and let it be good/done enough. One way to do this is to set a time to end your day, and at that point take a moment to jot down any outstanding tasks. Let this list be the starting point for the following day. It helps your mind to know you have those tasks written down, and also to know you can let them go for the evening and rest. Then, at the bottom of your list, inscribe this simple phrase: *The day is done. I accept it as it is.* In my (Diana's) house, when I do this practice, I also yell out to my family, "The day is done and the kitchen is CLOSED!"

Tips for Parental Detachment

Just because you love your kids doesn't mean you will always enjoy parenting. Cleaning out backpacks, signing school waivers, and dealing with tantrums isn't always fun. But if you find yourself detaching from your kids and yourself as a result, it's important to pause and find ways to reattach again. Detachment is a vicious cycle, because the more detached you feel, the more likely you are to pull away, which leads to more detachment. And the more detached you are, the more you will miss out on the wonderful aspects of parenting—like hugs, watching them grow, and feeling like you matter.

Often parents see parenting as a one-way street—it's your job to take care of your kids and make sure they are happy. But in reality, parenting is two-way. Your kids feel better when you are engaged; they want you to be fulfilled just as much as you want them to be happy. And when you are both doing well, you exchange this positive energy with each other! Try taking the perspective of your kids. What do you think it's like to have you as a parent? From behind their eyes, do they see you as living fully and with vitality? From their perspective, can you see that they want you to be happy just as much as you want them to be happy? Now, with this broader perspective in mind, make more room to do what you love with your kids (not just what they love).

Many parents find themselves shuttling their kids to various after-school activities while setting aside their own interests and movement needs. What if you were to design some after-school enrichment that enriches you too? If you love soccer, invite your kids to join you in kicking the ball around the yard; if you have a penchant for weight lifting, ask your kids to serve as a human barbell while you do some squats. Ultimately, what your children crave most is spending time with you, especially when you're in a less-stressed state. How you do this will change as your kids get older. When my (Diana's) boys were babies, I pushed them in a stroller on my favorite bike path; now I'm trail running with my teenager as he mountain bikes, and walking as my younger son horseback rides. I love to be outside with them, on the trail (that's my thing), but now they can each do their favorite thing too. Find things that you, not just your kids, love, and you both will benefit.

And be present with them while you do it. Instead of using every minute of your day to "get something done," be with your kids, or make getting something done secondary to being present. Let some things go, remembering that this time is short. What really matters here? Which leads to the next burnout dilemma…feeling ineffective.

Tips for Feelings of Ineffectiveness

If you care a lot about being a parent (which most parents do!), you are likely to set high standards for yourself. And because parenting is so challenging, this can lead us to often feeling like we are falling short. If you feel like you have to tackle everything on your own and are self-critical when you don't meet your standards, you are going to burn out.

This is where self-compassion can really help. Research shows that parents who are self-compassionate are better able to manage the stress of parenting. Try applying the three components of self-compassion: mindfulness, kindness, and common humanity. Mindfulness here might mean just checking in with yourself throughout the day and asking what you need (even if you can't give yourself what you need, acknowledging you have needs helps!). Instead of comparing yourself to other parents or wishing things to be different, just say to yourself, *Hey, how are you doing? Is there anything you need physically or emotionally right now?* Kindness involves speaking to yourself with the same kind of understanding and loving tone you would use when caring for your kids. *It's understandable you don't have energy to exercise; you are working hard at raising two young kids! Look at how much you ran around already today. Are there movements that would feel nourishing to you and that don't take much time?* And common humanity is remembering that millions of parents are in the same boat. This is hard, and you are not alone. You can practice self-compassion anywhere; it doesn't take any kind of special essential oil to treat yourself with self-compassion, it just takes remembering to be mindful, kind, and connected. Bring this mindfulness, kindness, and connection into your physical activity, and it can be a resource for you to reconnect.

Finally, parents are not meant to do it all alone. If you are unable to keep up with the daily demands of making meals and caring for your children, get some support. Get your kids involved in housework—it gives them a feeling of accomplishment and that they matter—and remember that they are learning so it's not going to be perfect. Also, enlist friends to trade childcare, and get creative with communal exchanges. For eons, human have leaned on alloparents—anyone who's not a biological parent of a child they're taking care of—to help raise their kids; it's beneficial for your children's development and your wellbeing. If you need a break and an exercise class away from your kids, see if you can trade with a friend!

Rethinking Movement
Focus, Energy, and Dynamic Rest

Fatigue is a feeling of extreme tiredness or lack of energy, and it can definitely impact how much you feel like exercising. While resting might always seem like you're listening to your body, depending on what type of fatigue you have—physical or attentional—moving your body might ultimately be the most *restorative* choice.

Physical fatigue develops when you've used up all your physical energy for the day, either using it all day, or maybe for a shorter period of time at a higher intensity. With mental fatigue, you can be mostly sedentary all day long and still feel exhausted from focusing your attention all day long. It's like your mind has been running on a treadmill without rest.

When you are physically fatigued, taking rest allows your body to respond by repairing and getting ready for the next day. When you are attentionally fatigued, you need a break from giving attention; you need *mental* downtime, and not necessarily the physical downtime that seems appealing. Especially if your downtime just consists of different forms of giving attention (like scrolling your phone or watching a show), consider a dose of *dynamic rest*.

Dynamic rest is just like it sounds: It's giving your attention muscles a break while you do something simple and repetitive with your body, like running, walking, cycling, swimming laps, or doing push-ups or spinal twists. It's letting a movement teacher guide you while you stop leading and just follow along. It's putting on your favorite music and dancing it out. Dynamic rest is a stack—of the movement *and* the type of rest you need.

Caring for children (of any age!) all day takes lots of focus, as does working on focused projects or spending a lot of time on email, texting, and other digital media. If you're feeling exhausted at the end of the day, take a moment to consider which type of exhaustion you have and what response would ultimately be your best use of time…and choose your next move accordingly.

Reason 15: I spend so much time and energy doing all the things I "have to" do: keeping the house, yard, self, etc. looking culturally acceptable. In other words, prioritizing spending my time on other things. I know what's best for me, but I frequently lose sight of it.

There is a cognitive bias in psychology called the Mere Urgency Effect, where individuals prioritize tasks that feel urgent over those that are more important but may not have an immediate time constraint. This can lead us to focus more time on the have-tos, while neglecting more meaningful stuff even when it has a significant long-term impact. It sounds like that is what is happening for you. You are lost in the weeds of all the "other things" and have lost track of using your time in ways that are best for you. The question is, then, how can you tune in to what's best for you and prioritize movement, even when everything else is screaming at you that it is urgent?

This is going to take some pausing and checking in throughout your day. By taking a mindful pause, you can get present and redirect your attention back to what is, as you say, "best for you." Mindfulness is paying attention to the present moment, with all your senses and without judgment. When you put some mindful pauses into your day, you can use them as opportunities to center yourself and ask, *What's best for me here?* And, *How can I add some movement here?* There are many ways to add movement into pretty much any activity you do, even while looking culturally appropriate! For instance, I (Diana) often blow-dry my hair while doing calf stretches.

No one is mindful all the time, so it can be helpful to have something to remind you. What will cue you to take committed action and pause?

In our house we have a mindfulness bell on all of our devices that goes off every hour to remind us to take a mindful pause. When it rings, we stop, take a breath, and come back to the present moment. Even my dog is trained up on this bell to stop! Having that mindful pause, even if it's only ten seconds, is a great way to check in and see that you have a choice in how you are engaging with this moment. Any cue will work to remind you to do this. You could make your cue be every time your phone buzzes, or every time you get in the car, or every time you open your fridge. Whatever your cue, take a moment to pause, take in three slow breaths, and ask yourself, *What is best for me right now?*

If you would like to listen to me (Diana) guide you through a Mindful Pause, you can find one here: uphill-books.com/IKISresources

There are so many things to do and prioritize in life, and no one will ever find a perfect balance. That's not the goal. Finding a "good enough" balance of movement while tending to all your activities is good enough. So, practice a mindful pause, remember what's best for you, and see if you can add a more beneficial, meaningful movement into your long list of have-tos!

Rethinking Movement
"Have-Tos" and Have-Tos

There are many actual have-tos in life, and movement is one of them. Since you've already put "have to" in quotes in your initial question, we know you get the difference. "Have-tos" are also important, but are there any you can let go of to make space for movement?

Having a clean house is amazing, but is it something you can let go of a bit now and then? Leaving the bed unmade is harmless. If you do the dishes instead of take the jog, you're likely to feel bad about not getting the movement you want. But if you take the jog, you're likely to come back with more energy and also do the dishes anyway. Or, can you delegate a "have-to" so you can have both a run and a clean kitchen?

And once you've prioritized getting some physical activity that is meaningful to you and having time to yourself (another must!), you could try making both have-tos and "have-tos" more densely packed with movement nutrients. Feel you have to clean right now? Ditch the power mop and get down on all fours to scrub the floor to fit in some harder core and arm movement; use a push mower instead of a riding one and there's your cardio; walk to get the groceries. The way our near ancestors got their have-tos done gave them way more movement, and this is part of why we often hear people say "my grandparents never exercised." There is a lot of movement to be found in the course of a normal day of responsibilities, and you can choose a few areas where you can complete a task in a way that moves you well. (But still go for that jog/walk/class/dance, ya hear?)

3

I'm Too Embarrassed

In psychology, embarrassment is an emotional response you have when you think you've made a mistake or violated social norms. Often when we feel embarrassed, it's accompanied by feeling self-conscious and wanting to hide or fix the situation. It's thought to be a good thing in some ways—it provides internal/societal feedback that helps keep us from repeating a mistake—but if we don't do things because we are embarrassed, then it becomes a barrier. It gets glitchy when we play it safe because we fear we will "die of embarrassment." Have you ever heard of anyone "dying" of embarrassment? Sure, you get sweaty palms, you feel a little flushed, your heart rate goes up, and then…you don't die. All emotion rises and falls. But we relate to it as if it is going to last forever.

Shame is a little different. It's deeper, more intense, and we feel it when we think there is something fundamentally wrong with us, not just that we made a mistake. Embarrassment tends to be focused on a specific event (e.g., you worry that people will notice that you get a red face when you exercise), whereas shame lingers and impacts how you view yourself as a person (e.g., you feel that you are a freak of nature because you get a red face when you exercise). Shame can lead to feelings of unworthiness, and is often linked to your overall self-worth. Shame often has its roots in trauma and negative learning history, and if you are experiencing it, you may benefit from working with a mental health professional.

The exercise landscape is just full of potential sources for embarrassment! *What if I'm dressed wrong? What if I don't know how to use the equipment? What if I'm the slowest or clumsiest one?* If you ask us, the gym and middle school kind of seem similar! Both are associated with big feelings, especially the fear that others might evaluate us negatively.

Physical activity can make us feel especially exposed and vulnerable to negative evaluation. Movement involves our bodies and all their parts and functions. Gross! It often includes going into spaces we're not familiar with, being with people we're not familiar with, and figuring out a lot of things on our own without much support. Like we said, middle school. Ew!

When we're afraid of judgement, we're ultimately afraid that we don't belong. When we're afraid to be judged by how we're moving, we're ultimately afraid we don't belong amongst other movers. But of course, this belief is heavily influenced by our own thoughts.

While we couldn't help you out in middle school, we've got your back this time around. To help you with embarrassment, we've included strategies to overcome barriers such as negative body image, body shame, fear of being judged by others, and social stigma. You will apply the principles of psychological flexibility to develop greater body-image flexibility, capitalize on the benefits of moving with others, and get more flexible with your embarrassing thoughts.

Embarrassment is so very tied up with societal convention, you can learn to approach movement from outside of the box, to chart your own path, and to be bold, even when it might feel embarrassing at first.

You already belong to a group of movers: you're a human being! Movement is for every body, and that includes yours.

Reason 16: When I move it makes me feel fat. My body jiggles, my thighs touch. I'm ashamed of my body and don't want to be reminded of it.

Welcome to having a human body in a society that does not celebrate the diversity of human bodies. Our bodies jiggle, they are squishy, they are crooked, they are all sorts of things, and they almost never match the picture of Instagram thigh gaps or flat abs. In today's culture, we are inundated with relentless fat-shaming messages saying there is something wrong with us if our body does not fit an unrealistic thin/fit ideal. Much of this messaging is designed to make us feel bad about our body so that we will buy something to fix it. Over time, we can internalize these messages along with negative messaging from our family and friends, and end up hating our bodies and avoiding moving them.

Before we offer you some ideas for getting more flexible with your body image and your movement, let's take a look at how body shame is impacting your behavior. What things are you doing to avoid or hide your body, and what are the consequences? This can open the door to asking yourself, is it worth it? And what do you want to do instead?

The Cost of Body Avoidance

Skipping physical activity helps you "forget" about your body and maybe avoid some embarrassment in the short term, but what do you miss out on when you take this approach? Answer the following in your notebook.

- When I avoid physical activity, my energy levels are…
- When I avoid physical activity, it impacts my relationships by…
- When I avoid physical activity, it impacts my work by…

- When I avoid physical activity, my mood is…
- When I avoid physical activity my embarrassment in the long run is…(worse/better/the same)

Consider some of the other ways you hide or avoid your body. Get curious. What are the costs to your energy, relationships, work, and mental health? Get out your notebook, label this page *Body Avoidance,* and answer these questions:

Clothing. Do you disguise or cover up your body through clothes? Do you wear uncomfortable clothes or not allow yourself to purchase clothes that you would enjoy wearing because of negative body image? What are you missing out on because of this avoidance?

Social activities. Do you avoid social situations that involve eating or moving or that focus on appearance? Do you avoid exercise classes, swimming, dancing, running, or walking with other people because you are ashamed of your body? What do you miss out on because of this avoidance?

Checking behaviors. Do you spend a lot of time or energy scrutinizing yourself in the mirror, measuring or weighing yourself, or otherwise checking on certain parts of your body? Do you use checking to avoid uncomfortable feelings and thoughts about your shape and weight? What are you missing out on because of this avoidance?

Intimacy. Do you hide your body from your partner, avoid intimacy, or avoid getting into a romantic relationship because of your negative body image? What are you missing out on because of this avoidance?

Physical activity. Do you avoid engaging in physical activities that remind you of your body, even when alone? What feelings or thoughts do physical activities elicit in you? What do you do to avoid these thoughts and feelings? What are you missing out on because of this avoidance?

Jiggle It Just a Little Bit (Or a Lot)

Body-image flexibility is your ability to embrace the present moment, including a negative body image, while pursuing your life values. That means that even if you have negative body image thoughts and feelings (which many of us do), you choose to move anyway!

With body-image flexibility, you can notice your jiggly thighs and "feeling fat," accept those as part of your current experience, and shift your attention and energy towards your movement goals and values. Here are two exercises you can try to build more body-image flexibility:

Perspective practice in the mirror. Set aside a few minutes when you can be alone and undisturbed. Position yourself in front of a mirror, giving yourself some space to comfortably view your reflection.

1. Shift your perspective. Instead of zeroing in on specific body parts, start by gazing at your entire body as if it were a panoramic view. Look at your body with the curiosity you might feel when taking in a vast landscape.

2. Embrace the whole picture. Focus on your body as a complete entity, appreciating its entirety rather than being critical of its individual features.

3. Look at your body for its function. How will this body help you move through your day today, complete what you need to get done, or express yourself?

4. Watch for over-focus. Be mindful of any tendency to hone in on one particular body part or aspect. When you notice your attention narrowing in this way, gently redirect it outward to the broader, holistic view of your body.

5. Practice with patience. Body-image flexibility is a skill that takes time. Be patient with yourself as you learn to see your body as an integrated whole. Take this practice with you into your day: When you catch yourself zooming in on one part you don't like, zoom back out again. And focus on function over form.

Embrace the jiggle. Acceptance doesn't mean you have to like your body or abandon your efforts for improvement. Instead, it's about embracing the challenging thoughts and uncomfortable feelings or sensations that may arise as you pursue what truly matters to you, such as connecting socially, fostering intimacy, or staying physically active.

1. Choose an activity you really want to do, even if it makes your body jiggle and triggers those "I feel fat" thoughts. Actually, if it *is* an extra-jiggly activity, you'll get more bang for your buck with this practice.

2. Before diving in, remind yourself why this activity is important to you. Is it your ticket to being more socially engaged, important to your physical health or pain management, something you enjoy, a way to be closer with your partner, or a way to be more connected to a hobby or sport you love?

3. Get willing. Deliberately let your body jiggle and wiggle as you engage in this activity. In fact, dial it up! How much jiggle can you make? Accept those jiggles and welcome any uncomfortable thoughts and feelings that come along for the ride. As you do, remind yourself, *I welcome this jiggly sensation because I value* _____.

4. Try including at least one extra-jiggly activity a week. The more you practice accepting the jiggle, the more flexible you are becoming. As it gets easier for you, you can increase the challenge by jiggling in public, jiggling in clothes that show your jiggle, jiggling with others. Go to your list of ways in which you hide your body and choose a few of them to try jiggling in. Remember that when you embrace the jiggle, you are freeing yourself to move, and you are also freeing yourself from fat-shaming culture. It's an act of body-image activism. All bodies deserve to move without shame or embarrassment.

Jiggly exercises

If you're wondering what movements you might add to get you jiggling once a week, here are some ideas to get you started!

Jump rope, bounce on a rebounder, shimmy, twerk, battle rope, have a kitchen dance party, do box jumps, play hopscotch, use a hula hoop, run up some stairs, run down a hill, take a belly-dancing class.

Movement Reframe
The Way It Looks, the Way It Works

So your thighs touch. What else can they do? Do they get you in and out of chairs? Carry you up and down stairs? Keep your head above water when you're swimming? Help you shake your booty when dancing?

So your body jiggles. What else can it do? Can it ride a bike? Does it get you from point A to point B all day, every day? Move you around for work and chores? Give a great hug? Sing beautifully?

Body appreciation is the ability to accept, respect, and have gratitude for your physical form, regardless of its physical appearance. Research shows that the more body-appreciative you are, the easier it is to choose to move. When you respect your body, you're more apt to take care of its needs, and movement is one of its needs!

To transition away from a "the way it looks" mindset to a "the way it works" one, take out your journal and note all the ways your body is working for you.

- Which parts are strong?

- Which parts feel good?

- Which parts work pain-free all the time, and never get any credit?

Exercise is often paired with language about the way we look. Don't like how your body looks now? Exercise. Want to keep enjoying the way your body looks? Exercise. Despite all the benefits that have nothing to do with appearance (improved mood, strength, skill, stamina, protection from disease, etc.), exercise's appearance-rich framing continues to persist in many realms, but those realms don't have to include your own mind.

While your body isn't a machine, for many folks, thinking of the body as a series of parts coming together to work in a way that keeps us alive and engaged can be a helpful tool. Movement greases the joints, and reinforces the scaffolding that holds us up and the pulleys that articulate our parts.

Reason 17: I want to go walking with friends, but I'm out of shape. So I don't go when they ask.

It's great that you want to walk with friends. It sounds like feeling out of shape is making you hesitant to join them. It's really common for us to compare ourselves to others, fear that they will judge us, and shy away from joining in if we think we're going to fall behind. It kind of brings us back to being in school, doesn't it? To those times we didn't make the team, or someone laughed at us for running too slow, or blamed us for losing the game. Or when our gym teacher wrote everyone's time on the board and we were close to last. Neither of us will ever forget the anxiety we used to feel before having to run the timed mile in grade school!

Before offering some tips to work with comparison, let's highlight why it's not a good idea to let comparison steal this social experience from you, and why walking with your friends is so good for you.

Benefits of Moving with Others

Friends are a psychological resource. Exercising with friends can change how you perceive physical challenges, and moving with friends gives you extra boost in energy. For example, in a study called "Social Support and the Perception of Geographical Slant," researchers found that when participants had a friend with them, they estimated a hill as less steep than when they were alone. The longer they'd known the friend, the less steep they perceived the hill! In a second study described in the same paper, just the thought of supportive friends made participants perceive the hill as less steep. These researchers described friends as a valuable "psychological resource" for facing difficult physical challenges. Walking with friends may actually make walking less daunting, especially if you are feeling "out of shape." (And make sure you pick your best friends for the biggest hills!)

You'll perform better than you expect. There's a phenomenon in psychology called the Köhler effect that suggests that when you perform a difficult task with someone who is slightly better than you, you perform better than you would alone. For example, in a study where research participants were asked to hold a plank position alongside another person whose performance was manipulated to always be superior to theirs, they persisted longer than when they held the plank on their own. In other words, walking with friends who are in slightly better shape than you just may up your performance. You may be able to walk longer or harder when you walk with stronger friends.

You're more likely to stick with it. Walking with others increases your sense of belonging, strengthens your bonds, builds accountability to a group, and can make your movement more enjoyable. A review of research studies published in the *Journal of Preventive Medicine* found that people who exercised with others had long-term adherence rates of almost 70 percent. You want to show up because your friends depend on you and it's fun to move with others.

It's good for your brain. Exercising with others also gives you an extra brain boost. According to Dr. Jenny Etnier, a researcher in kinesiology at the University of North Carolina, when you combine physical activity with socializing, it engages your memory and attention, promoting the formation of vital connections between brain cells and keeping your thinking skills sharp. You will be building social connection and neuronal connections at the same time!

Overcoming Social Comparison

You said you want to go walking with friends, but being out of shape is your barrier. Let's use some psychological flexibility skills to help you get over the social-comparison hump so that you can start doing what you want to do (and what is great for you).

Don't trust your mind's bad advice. It's human to want to belong to a group, but the advice our mind gives us to fit in often leads us to feel more alone. For example, your mind may be telling you things like, *They* *will judge me, Everyone else is fitter than me,* or *I can't tell them how I really feel.* What does your mind say when you think about going for a walk with friends? Are your thoughts helpful or demotivating? Use your cognitive flexibility skills. Observe these as just thoughts, and instead of listening to this bad advice, you can say, "Thank you, mind," and let them go. Redirect your behavior towards what you want to do: Walk with friends. If your mind is giving you bad advice, spot it, thank it, but don't follow it!

What do you really want? Next, check in with your deepest values. Why is moving with your friends important to you? Review some of the benefits above. Which ones resonate with you? Do you care about feeling challenged? Do you care about social support? Do you care about your brain health? Remind yourself of these values when you are headed out for a walk, instead of listening to your mind's resistance.

Be honest with your friends. The best way to build connections is through vulnerable, authentic conversations. In fact, research shows that revealing personal, vulnerable information doesn't make others judge us— it makes them like us more! When we share our vulnerable secrets with others, they see us as more honest and trustworthy.

Talk to your friends about your concerns. They might not even be aware that you're struggling. Tell them you are afraid you're out of shape, you won't keep up, or you'll hold them back. Honest communication can lead to greater understanding, and they can work with you to generate some creative solutions. For example, you can alternate who sets the pace for the group, or find stopping points along the way where you can meet up. You may be surprised how well your friends respond when you're vulnerable, and you might even find that they sometimes feel the same way.

We all have parts of ourselves we feel embarrassed about, we compare, and we fear don't measure up. For example, I (Diana) am pretty inexperienced at water sports, although I love the water. So for years I avoided getting on a surfboard or paddleboard out of fear of looking like a beginner. Well, guess what! That meant I stayed a beginner. When I finally stopped listening to my mind's bad advice and tried it out, I had a really hard time popping up (getting into a standing position on the board)! As was to be expected. But when I showed a video to a few friends, they didn't see it as a failure, they saw it as being brave.

Focus your attention on meaningful conversation. If you aren't focusing on your mind's bad advice, what should you focus on? Something much more interesting—your friends! Not only does engaging conversation enhance the cognitive benefits of exercise, it can also increase your feeling of belonging and connection. You may want to try out some of these questions that have been scientifically shown to increase closeness. Here's some conversation starters to use on your walk:

- What would constitute a "perfect" day for you?
- For what in your life do you feel most grateful?
- If you could wake up tomorrow having gained any quality or ability, what would it be?

Take committed action. We've presented a lot of research here demonstrating why walking with friends is great for you, and how you can use psychological flexibility skills to help you do it. But ultimately you are your own best judge. Be a scientist and set up a little self-experiment! Plan on going for at least two walks this week—one with friends and one alone. After each walk, record your answers to these questions in your notebook under the title *Is Walking With Friends Beneficial To Me?*

- Was my walk with friends or alone?
- How did this walk impact my mood?
- How did this walk impact my ability to pay attention and think creatively?
- How much energy did I have on this walk? How hard was it for me?
- Do I feel more or less connected to others?

The results of your test may be the best motivator yet. And, if you end up feeling worse after your walk with friends, you also may want to take a look at who you're calling friends! Choose people who are energizing, supportive, accepting, and growth oriented like you. And tell them what you are up to in working through this book. They may have their own barriers to movement that they need help with.

What's most important is that you and your values, not your mind's judgements, get to choose how you move and who you move with.

Rethinking Movement
All Sorts of Walking Buddies

Everybody has their own walking pace and everyone will have different paces throughout their lifetime, not only because we age, but because we all cycle through fitness and energy levels, and we all experience illness and injury. Thus, being out of step with others' walking pace is bound to happen sometimes. Does this mean you have to walk alone? Nope.

As we've already said, you can communicate with your friends about your specific needs. Invite them on a walk that works for you. Try texting the group: "I'm feeling like my energy is low today, but I want to get outside and move. Is anyone up for an easy-paced twenty-minute walk around the park this evening?" Or maybe: "I want to work on my endurance, and am currently clocking a thirty-minute mile. Anyone want to join me tomorrow morning? (Wear a rucksack if you want to bump up your intensity without leaving me behind!)"

Another approach is to find a walking partner who matches up with your current walking pace. Get all the benefit of walking with others, even if they're not your good friends (yet). There are likely walking or hiking groups in your area that go the distances or paces that work for you right now. Maybe there are people in your workplace keen to take a gentle, non-sweaty walk every day at lunchtime.

When I (Katy) was healing a fractured foot, I wasn't able to do the longer and faster walks my friends and I were used to. But still, I walked! I asked my walking friends whether they'd be up for a short, slow walk for some nature-rich, dynamic hangout time. Other times, I reached out to my so-called "non-walking" friends. I was surprised to find these friends were happy to join me on slower, shorter walks—it turns out that they had just been feeling too "out of shape" for the faster group! Now with a fully healed foot, I've doubled my number of walking friends, and thus my walks. Some are fast and some are slow, some are long and some are short. All are with friends, all are enjoyable, and every one makes me feel better.

Reason 18: I was raised in purity culture, where we were taught that being too sensual/sexual was wrong. I never felt completely comfortable or free in a public setting to do stretches, squats, any kind of dancing, or anything that may draw attention to my body.

Family, religious, or social moral codes can really interfere with our feeling free to move. When we are taught that moving our body equates to being sensual/sexual, and that being sensual/sexual is wrong, it can lead to feelings of shame or self-consciousness while exercising. If we learned these messages during adolescence—a pivotal time in our identity development—they can be extra hard to shake. Let's identify the beliefs you want to get more flexible around, and choose more compassionate self-talk, as you reclaim the freedom to move your body.

The Purity Patrol

Begin by exploring the beliefs about your body and movement that stem from your upbringing. Some beliefs you hold might include the following:

- Your body is sinful or shameful.
- Your body is out of control and makes you want things you shouldn't want.
- You must avoid drawing attention to your body.
- You should trust other people's opinions about your body over your own.
- Your body is dangerous.
- Pleasure is bad.

Take a walk and reflect on your experience, or walk and talk with a friend. What messages have you internalized about your body and movement? Whose voices do you hear in your head when it comes to moving your body? Who is the "purity patrol" still policing how you carry yourself? Your parents? A teacher? A religious or political figure? A family member? A TV show, book, or other media?

When you return, get out your notebook and make a list of the rules those voices tell you. You can title this *The Purity Patrol*. As you write the rules, identify the voice that goes with each. This helps with developing your own perspective, separate from theirs. For example:

- You can't wear tight clothes or show your skin. (Grandfather)
- You can't stretch your legs wide if people are looking. (Teacher)
- You can't dance in public. (Church)
- You can't do squats in those shorts. (Mom)

It may be impossible to erase these voices from your mind altogether, especially if you heard them at a young age. However, by naming the purity patrol as voices other than your own, you begin to get a little space from them. With this space that you can start to claim your own self-compassionate voice.

Compassionate Self-Talk

Imagine you could go back in time and meet yourself when you were first learning some of these beliefs about your body. Picture yourself at that age, how you felt about yourself, what you loved to do, and what you wished you would have heard. In your notebook, label a page *Compassionate Self-Talk* and answer some of these questions.

- What would you tell yourself about your body?
- What would you tell yourself about pleasure?
- What would you tell yourself about movement and play?

- What tone of voice would you use towards yourself?

For example:

You are the authority on your body. You can trust and respond to your body's needs and desires. You can enjoy your body, move it, and are free to express yourself in it. You are safe in your own body.

Once you have a compassionate message to offer your younger self, try offering it to yourself now. When you are moving your body and the purity patrol shows up, take on the facial expression of your most compassionate wise self (see pages 33–35) and remind yourself that you can choose a different way of relating to your body from the one you were taught.

Seek Community and Support

Healing from purity culture often requires the help of others. You may want to consider seeking a therapist who specializes in trauma, online support groups, or books for more support. For example: *Educated* by Tara Westover, *Pure: Inside the Evangelical Movement That Shamed a Generation of Young Women and How I Broke Free* by Linda Kay Klein, or *Come as You Are: The Surprising New Science that Will Transform Your Sex Life* by Emily Nagoski.

Rethinking Movement
Movement is Biological and Cultural

So much about the way we move is biological—the shape of our joints, the length of our bones, the stretchiness of our nerves. And at the same time, the cultures we exist in also impact the way we move. For women especially, the additional cultural barriers can be tremendous. Researchers are looking to figure out why the women in some places are so inactive and have found families or partners discouraging the act of exercise itself. Beliefs that workout clothing is "inappropriate," sport is a men's activity, and exercise might harm reproduction are just some of the reasons physical activity is discouraged. For others, being mobile in daily life—simply heading out for a walk—can be seen as a suggestive and thus unsafe activity.

Some research has found correlations between religiosity and pelvic floor disorders like chronic pelvic pain and pain with intercourse in women. (Finding a physical therapist that specializes in pelvic floor therapy can be so helpful when it comes to dealing with this!)

Other research has shown that the problem is not religiosity so much as any messaging that sex is bad. The impact of this messaging on pelvic floor issues is not necessarily limited to women; it could also be impacting male bodies, but there's just a dearth of research on male pelvic floor disorder overall, and no investigations into how it's affected by purity culture...yet!

Even in cultures outside of these extremes, many women hunch their spines to mask their breasts or skip higher-impact movement all together—not for the physical discomfort of moving breasts, but because of the attention they feel this movement might bring. I (Katy), who focused on pelvic floor disorders in graduate school, heard time and time again from the women I worked with that they were explicitly taught to tuck their bottoms under for modesty's sake, and had been actively clenching this area for decades, almost subconsciously!

If you've discovered other voices in your head that are moving your body in ways you don't want them to anymore, work on reconnecting yourself to the *biology* of movement. While sex is biological, it's just one thing our body does among hundreds of other things. Right now the voices in your head saying these common, everyday movements are sexualized are louder than your own voice. For every movement you want to do, think of two or three ways it serves a need you have so *your* voice is the loudest. *I'm squatting instead of sitting in a chair so my lower back feels good the rest of the day, to stretch my hips so I can walk farther tomorrow, and to fit in my daily exercise because I can't get to the gym later. Or: I'm dancing because I love this song, I'm fitting in some physical activity while also being at this wedding, and it's so fun to connect with my friends in this moment."*

Reason 19: I feel judged when I try to fit in some exercise while waiting around in public spaces–especially those where the expectation is that you should just be sitting there.

Achieving and maintaining good health in a culture where a sedentary lifestyle is the norm often requires deviating from the usual path. Most of our spaces are designed to favor sitting, so it's no wonder most public settings—airports, schools, sports venues, and meeting rooms—cue us to be sedentary. People might see you as weird when you choose to pace, stand, stretch, squat, or fidget in these spaces, simply because you're behaving differently from how everyone was expecting.

Be a Healthy Deviant

In her book *The Healthy Deviant*, Pilar Gerasimo introduces the term *healthy deviant* to describe someone who consciously breaks away from unhealthy societal norms to achieve higher resilience, vitality, and autonomy. In these times in our society, the straightforward, readily available, and default choice often leads to a sedentary lifestyle and unhealthy outcomes. According to Gerasimo, following the default path will likely result in a decline in your health and happiness over time. We need to deviate! Challenging cultural norms in a society that promotes unhealthy habits is necessary for us to properly care for ourselves.

That being said, stepping away from the norm can cause anxiety for many of us. Humans have evolved to be part of groups and avoid standing out. It can be uncomfortable (and sometimes dangerous) to be different. If you choose healthy deviance, you'll need to face some of your fears head-on.

Exposure

One effective way to get more flexible, even with anxiety, is through a technique commonly used in cognitive behavioral therapy approaches called *exposure*. Exposure is a psychological technique in which you gradually expose yourself to the feared object or situation. With ACT-based exposure, the goal isn't to get rid of your anxiety, but to become flexible with your behavior, even with anxiety present. The process involves making a hierarchy of fears from least feared to most, then moving up the ladder, one fear at a time, as you become increasingly flexible with them.

In the exercise below, you will use exposure to face your fear of deviating from social norms by moving into public spaces.

1. Create your hierarchy of social deviance. Get out your notebook and label the page *My Social Deviance Brainstorm.*

Begin by writing down the places where you'd like to incorporate more physical activity but it goes against the cultural norm. Then, get creative and brainstorm various activities you could engage in within these sedentary settings. Below are some ideas.

While watching TV:

- play a physical game with your kids
- install a pull-up bar and hang from it
- stretch during commercials
- remove furniture in front of screens
- install a climbing wall in your TV room

At work:

- offer walking meetings in your online calendar
- stand and fidget during online meetings
- take ten-minute movement breaks every hour
- use an exercise ball as a chair
- stretch at a wall during conferences

While traveling:

- walk in circles at the airport
- carry your rolling suitcase
- choose stairs over moving walkways, escalators, and elevators
- opt for walking instead of taking trams or shuttles
- squat while waiting in line

While cooking and eating meals:

- walk to a scenic spot for picnics
- walk or bike to restaurants or dessert places
- enjoy a family walk after dinner
- squat while eating or preparing food
- get rid of chairs and sit on the floor
- whisk cream, chop veggies, grind coffee, shell nuts by hand

During kids' activities:

- walk or jog around the sports field during games
- cross the bars, slide on the slide, walk the bouncy bridge with your kids
- stand outside bleachers and stretch
- sit and stretch on the ground instead of bringing your travel chair
- coach sports teams or practice with kids
- sign up kids for parent/child dance, music, or fitness classes

2: Rank your activities. Pick ten activities that are most linked to your values. Next draw a ladder on the page. List the activities that are most intimidating at the top of the ladder and work your way down to least intimidating at the bottom, as we've demonstrated. This is your hierarchy of deviance.

High fear:

- offer walking meetings on my online calendar
- stand during meetings
- squat while waiting in line
- carry my rolling suitcase
- sit on a ball at work
- stretch while watching my kid's sports games

Low fear:

- carry grocery bags in arms out of the grocery store instead of using a cart
- stay standing on the bus even if there are empty seats
- enjoy a family walk after dinner
- stretch during commercials

3. Move up your ladder one rung at a time. Start at the bottom of your list and pick one activity to try first. Keep repeating the behavior until you feel more flexibility around it. Again, the fear may not go away, but you may get better at having the fear and doing the activity anyway. Practice acceptance as you do it, opening up to the fear with your mind, body, and behavior. Then work your way up.

Commit to practicing at least three healthy deviant behaviors each week. As you become more flexible with the activities lower on the list, increase the level of challenge, and eventually do as many as possible.

As you engage in your healthy deviant behaviors, allow for thoughts that you are being judged or getting weird looks from others. Embrace this experience as part of being a healthy deviant and refocus your attention on your movement values. You can also enhance your accountability by inviting a friend to join you in socially deviant activities or sharing your experiences on social media. Finding a community of other healthy deviants helps you feel empowered by challenging the default unhealthy reality.

Remember, when you step out of your comfort zone and incorporate movement into traditionally sedentary spaces, you may encounter some curious looks, but you might also find unexpected companions. Your courage to move your body can inspire and grant permission to others to do the same.

Rethinking Movement
Permission to Move, Granted

One way to change a sedentary culture is to simply behave differently yourself. Another way is to change the environment to make it easier for others to move too.

In spaces where you have greater impact on the movement culture, grant everyone permission to move. If you run team gatherings at work, let people know at the beginning of the meeting that they're welcome to stand or stretch at the edge of the room, and have a few clipboards handy for their note-taking. Bring a couple of blankets to the sidelines at soccer games or other gatherings and invite people to sit on the ground with you. I (Katy) have created signs to post in homes, classrooms, and offices that signal where kids CAN jump and twirl and get their wiggles out. (Find a link to these free downloads in the resources section.)

I've also been working on a simple series of "stretching here is welcome" signs and I'm approaching airports (many of which already have playground spaces for kids) to see if they'll install them in certain areas to give more people permission/encouragement to move their bodies before long stretches of air-travel immobility.

In a culture where sedentarism is the norm and the "polite" behavior, we have to get explicit when it comes to encouraging ourselves and others to shift the needle.

Reason 20: At twenty-four years old, I was a competitive swimmer/runner/football player. Now forty years old, I compare myself to the athlete I was then and it makes me feel like a loser. I will never be that in shape again, and every time I get started with an exercise program I am reminded of that.

When you've been a competitive athlete, it can become a part of your identity. But when we over-identify with one aspect of ourselves, we can get rigid in our view. We think there is only one way to be an athlete, and that if we are not that way, we aren't measuring up. Or we believe that our worth is based on our athletic performance, and we bail on doing activities because we have set such high expectations for ourselves. But no matter what story you tell yourself about who you were, or who you are, it does not capture all of you. You are so much more than the story your mind is creating about you. And the story your mind is creating is keeping you from letting your inner athlete, and all your other inner qualities (goofball? Adventurer? Friend? Teammate?) shine. Let's take a broader, wiser perspective on you than the "either/or" story your mind is drumming up: *I am either a "competitive athlete" or a "loser."*

Your history of being an athlete has likely impacted you in positive ways that are still with you—like having stamina, being a team player, predicting what might come next, or bouncing back after a loss. Instead of basing your worth on a fixed sense of self (your peak performance sixteen years ago), try seeing yourself with a bigger lens. You are a human whose body and strengths are in a constant state of change and evolution.

You can step back from your "loser" mentality and use this wiser perspective to support the movement habits you're trying to build.

A Wise View

Answer these questions in your notebook under the title *My Wise Athlete Self*:

- What strengths did you cultivate as a competitive athlete that can now support your efforts to regain fitness? For instance, did your sports experiences build qualities like persistence, grit, collaboration, or leadership?

- What wisdom have you gained from transitioning out of being a competitive athlete? What have you learned about your ability to adapt to change? Or what have you learned about what's important to you beyond being just an athlete? How can you lean on this wisdom when you think you are a loser?

- Expand your perspective across time. If you were to meet your athlete self sixteen years ago, what advice would you give them about physical activity and caring for their body? And if you were to meet yourself sixteen years from now, what advice would your older self give you about caring for yourself and your body?

This wise view can help you out when you're feeling blocked around exercise and physical activity. When the story shows up that you are a loser, remind yourself that you have many parts that have evolved and changed over time—you still have an athlete within that you can lean on to help you get moving, and you also have a wise part that embraces change, sees your many strengths, and wants the best for you now. Use this wise view to help you out. You are more than the story your mind is telling you.

Rethinking Movement
What does a Forty-Eight-Year-Old Athlete Look Like?

I (Katy) am going to be a tough-love coach for you right now. What if the way you're feeling doesn't stem from the fact that you're not the athlete you used to be at twenty-four, but because you're not the athlete you could be at forty?

Research on athletic identity and physical activity level after "retirement" from competitive play shows that former college athletes don't engage in more physical activity than non-athletes. Why not? These are folks who allotted a tremendous volume of time to training and practice (sticking to a program isn't a problem for them, obviously), are aware of their bodies and how to develop strength and skill, and feel like they belong in movement spaces. So why don't they continue to be active at a greater rate than those who aren't starting off with such a great "prepared to exercise" list? The answer seems to be tied up with identity. Athletes aren't engaged in physical training for the sake of their health and wellness. Instead, athletes are motivated by becoming better at their sport, or by competition. Most exercise programs lack these elements and don't align with an "athlete" identity. In this case, you have some options: Learn to value regular ol' working out for what it is and can do for you, or pick a movement plan that features the sports you love playing and even some regular competition.

Once you've got a mode of movement figured out, you need to get real and deal with your age and stage. It's easier to be an athlete when you're younger, but it's not necessarily due to the *biology* of age. There's quite a bit of research on retired high-performance athletes because of the negative impact that changing up so many aspects of life—physical, social, and emotional—can have on them. Even for high school and college athletes, transitioning away from youth is hard, not because of changes to the physical body, but because of the loss of ample leisure time necessary for training. It's so much easier to stay in shape when we're younger; a full load of responsibilities haven't kicked in yet. When they do, training time is often downgraded to a handful of hours a week instead of the few hours each day that make up a younger athlete's movement diet. Being an athlete is also more externally rewarded when you're younger. When you're older, being an athlete is more about your relationship with yourself. When the fans are all gone, do you still want to play? If you do show up, you'll discover what it looks and feels like to be an older athlete, and whether you do indeed love sport or if you just loved being young.

This all said, there are plenty of older athletes. What they have in common is realistic goals for their performance (which *isn't the same* as expecting inevitable decline), regularly using psychological skills like positive self-talk (e.g., check in with your use of the invective *loser*), and putting their athlete's training to broader use by regularly pursuing challenging and meaningful goals—not only physical ones.

Part of maintaining (or regaining) your ability to be an athlete is to bear in mind that an athlete's physical training does not have to be—in fact, should not be—all sport. It's actually better to have a diverse movement diet that includes training, active recovery, mobility work, and other "movement supplements" that balance out the demands of your favorite ways of moving. But when it comes to motivation, remember it's not the playing that makes the athlete; it's a consistent need for self-improvement and competition (even against oneself) through physical performance. Instead of approaching exercise as a physical activity requirement, try meeting your need for self-improvement and competition instead and see how that makes you feel. Performance will always be relative to age, but getting into the flow, i.e., finding your athletic state in this case, will feel the same at every age: exhilarating!

Reason 21: I am in a larger-sized body and am tired of people telling me I am not "healthy" at this size and shape. I would love to try yoga to manage my stress, but it is another place where I feel like I don't fit in. The people who walk out of yoga studios don't look like me, and I feel judged by them.

Although many yoga studios are making attempts to be more inclusive of body diversity, many still give out the vibe that you must be thin, white, flexible, and wearing the right outfit to do yoga. Not only is this message harmful, it's a misinterpretation of what yoga is. As Susanna Barkataki writes in *Embrace Yoga's Roots*, "We have made some mistakes and gotten confused in our practice of yoga in the West. The criteria for practicing yoga itself is quite simple. Anything not leading toward unity is not yoga."

At its roots, yoga is about union and connection, and it's disheartening that yoga studios have turned into places where you don't feel welcome. Here are some ways to reconnect with yourself, and others, so that you can use yoga in ways that are beneficial to you—to reduce stress and experience some peace in your mind and body.

Find a body-inclusive yoga class. It might take some effort and committed action, but finding a studio that embraces all bodies is worth it. There is a wide variety of yoga studios (some feel more like gyms, others like spiritual centers), and only you will know which one feels right for you. When searching for a class, use terms like *body-positive yoga, trauma-informed yoga*, or *yoga for all sizes*. You may want to go check out the studio ahead of time to see how you feel there. You can stop by without participating in a class and see if the atmosphere resonates with you. Additionally, ask for recommendations and look into instructors' social media and websites to see if they promote diversity in terms of body shapes, ages, colors, abilities, and sizes.

Engage with body-inclusive media. Research shows that following social media pages that celebrate body diversity can improve your body image. When women ages eighteen to twenty-four followed body-positive or body-neutral posts daily for fourteen days, they reported improved body satisfaction and less tendency to compare their appearance with others, compared to those who engaged in typical social media behaviors, including viewing appearance-focused or idealized content. These improvements were maintained for four weeks after viewing the content. Follow social media channels and read books geared towards body inclusivity. Some resources that might help: Jessamyn Stanley and her book *Every Body Yoga: Let Go of Fear, Get On the Mat, Love Your Body*; Sonya Renee Taylor and her book *The Body Is Not an Apology: The Power of Radical Self-Love*; and Susanna Barkataki and her book *Embrace Yoga's Roots: Courageous Ways to Deepen Your Yoga Practice*.

Practice at home. If the idea of a group class feels intimidating, consider practicing yoga at home. There are numerous online resources, including videos and apps, that offer guided yoga sessions you can do in the comfort and privacy of your own space. This allows you to develop your practice at your own pace without worrying about judgment. Some of my (Diana's) favorite inclusive, all-level online classes are at my home studio Yoga Soup, yogasoup.com.

Use yoga to improve your body image. It can be hard to feel excluded, and yet keep up a positive self-image. There's some emerging research that yoga can improve your body image—women who practice yoga have higher body-image satisfaction and greater awareness of their body sensations and are less likely to report negative body image and disordered eating. Plus, when used as an intervention, doing twelve weeks of yoga was shown to decreased internalized weight stigma and increase intuitive eating. Remember that yoga isn't just about poses and postures—its true roots are in the union between your body, mind, and soul. Here are some ways you can help focus your practice to improve your body image:

- Cultivate awareness of your body's internal sensations rather than fixating on its external appearance. When you are in class, notice what the pose feels like from the inside. Which parts of your body are tightest, most open? What does inner alignment feel like without looking in the mirror?

- Respond to your body's signals with respect, avoiding the urge to push it beyond its limits. Instead, collaborate with your body to gradually expand your flexibility. When you notice a tight spot, breathe into it, inviting it to release, but not forcing.

- Pay attention to how you feel emotionally in each pose. Some people notice feelings of empowerment in standing poses like warrior or mountain pose, or feel comforted and supported in forward-folding poses like child's pose or standing forward fold. Uses poses to express and support your emotions.

- Find equilibrium between effort and ease within each posture or movement. For example, when you are in downward dog, you can feel the strength of your palms on the ground, and long back, while also relaxing into and letting yourself rest in the pose. Yoga can be both at the same time.

- Practice self-compassion on your way to class, in class, and after class. Remember that your worth is not determined by your body size or shape. You are so much more than that! How can you use yoga to treat your body with the utmost care, love, and gentleness? It can be helpful to work with a therapist or counselor who specializes in body-image issues to address any underlying feelings of stigma or self-criticism.

Yoga is a personal practice, and I hope it can become a source of stress reduction and body connection for you. And I hope you can let it go, too, if it doesn't work for you! There are many ways to move your body; yoga isn't the be-all and end-all.

Rethinking Movement
The Many Ways to Yoga

There has never been a larger buffet of ways to learn movement than there is now, and that goes for yoga too! If you're not able to find a live, in-person class that feels like the right fit, there's likely a pre-recorded video program, weekly live online class, or book that will fit you to a T. We absolutely need major changes to make movement spaces more inclusive, but if you're not able to find that space right now, there's likely a way to still follow your intuition about the benefits yoga can have on your mental health and start getting that type of movement programming right now.

Reason 22: I can't help but compare myself to other people in my exercise class. I always feel like I am the least coordinated, slowest, weakest of the group. I don't want to feel that way, so I don't go.

All humans compare themselves. Social comparison has its roots in our evolutionary history. It was how we humans were able to navigate groups, assess our status, and maintain our belonging.

Social comparison in itself isn't a bad thing. Sometimes comparing ourselves to others can be motivating and help us set goals we didn't think we could achieve until we saw someone else do it. Think about all the times you have been inspired by seeing someone else being physically active: Simone Biles on the vault, your seventy-five-year-old mom taking a dance class, seeing someone do a cool strength-training move or stretch on Instagram. Social comparison can be motivating...if you are focusing on helpful aspects of it, and if you are allowing yourself to be your own unique expression of yourself.

There's a way to be uplifted around others in an exercise class—the energy and group comradery can be contagious—as long as you can separate from negative, self-judgmental thoughts that bring you down. This takes being present and developing what psychologists call *flexible attention*. Flexible attention is your capacity to shift your attention to where you want it to go, the way you shine a flashlight in the direction you want to walk. You may not be in control of what is happening in your exercise class, who shows up, or even your thoughts and feelings, but you can control your attention.

What Are You Paying Attention To?

Let's explore what you're paying attention to in class. Where are you shining your flashlight?

Here are some unhelpful things you may be paying attention to:

- your performance compared to others
- how weak you feel
- how you look in the mirror
- every time you miss a step
- your critical self-talk
- your speed compared to others
- thoughts that others are looking at you

Anything else that you want to add? Where is your attention when you are comparing yourself in a negative way?

Attention Training

The trick here is to use your skills of being present and having cognitive flexibility to shift your attention to more helpful things. Next time you are in your exercise class, bring your full attention to the aspects of class you want to amplify and be present with them.

You might turn your attention outward:

- the group moving together in synchrony
- someone in the group who has dynamic, positive energy
- the coordination skills of another exerciser that you want to learn from
- playful, fun, or energizing feelings of working out with others
- other people who aren't perfectly coordinated

Or you might turn your attention to your own inner experience:

- the sensation of your feet making contact with the ground, e.g., the lifting, moving, and placing of each foot
- the rhythm of the music
- your body making subtle adjustments to balance
- signs that you are working hard, like your heart beating, your breath, or heat in your body
- feelings of competence, growth, pride that you are stepping out of your comfort zone

Anything else you want to add?

Choose a few items from this list (or pick your own) and make a commitment to pay attention to them. If your mind wanders to negative criticism, say, "Thank you, mind," and shift it to what is helpful to you.

Check in with yourself after class. Did shifting your attention change your experience? What aspects of your exercise class were most helpful to pay attention to? How could you bring this flexible attention to other places where you move your body but tend to compare yourself?

Rethinking Movement
Who Is the Slowest?

So, there's definitely a benefit to strengthening your attention muscles so you can keep yourself from spiraling down the hole of shame and get back to that exercise class again and again. But once you've logged some attention-muscle reps, another muscle that might need a little flexing is the SO WHAT? muscle.

Even in the fastest group of humans, someone will be the slowest. Even amongst the most coordinated humans, someone will be the least coordinated. Even in the best-dressed group, there's going to be the person with the worst outfit. Why wouldn't it be you sometimes?

In fact, it certainly *will* be you sometimes, and sometimes it will be me (Katy), and sometimes it will be that guy over there. SO WHAT? Being the slowest or the least coordinated doesn't say anything about the value of movement nutrients you're getting in an exercise class, and it doesn't say anything about your value as a person. If you're auditioning for a dance squad, you might not make it. If you're running a race, you probably won't medal. But other than those scenarios, which probably weren't values or goals of yours anyway, self-evaluations like these are meaningless in the bigger picture. So you're slow. SO WHAT? So you're not as coordinated as you'd like. SO WHAT?

Thinking SO WHAT? is another way to practice cognitive flexibility. The person who is controlling the rules is you. When you say SO WHAT to your mind, you're showing up for yourself, which is always on time, always the right move, and never out of style.

4

It's Uncomfortable

It's human to want to feel comfortable. Physically, we want to be free from pain, get enough rest, have energy and enough food and water. Psychologically we want to feel calm, free of anxiety and stress, and in control of our environment. But what if our attempts to "get comfortable" are getting in the way of what we value?

Sometimes moving our bodies doesn't feel good (like those physical therapy exercises you need to do after surgery). And sometimes moving our bodies isn't the most psychologically comfortable either (like the embarrassment you feel when your body jiggles).

Sometimes the discomfort is physical, like joint pain, being too cold or hot, or feeling tired; other times the discomfort we experience is emotional, like feelings of anxiety, dread, grief, or the feelings that come with being told we *have* to do something (a lack of control!).

Whether physical or emotional, pushing yourself through discomfort does not usually work in the long run. Unfortunately, trying to avoid the discomfort that comes with physical activity doesn't work out in the long run either—our tissues require us to move, and when we don't, we significantly increase our chances of physical pain from injury and disease over time. So, there's discomfort either way, which is why our goal is not to *eliminate* discomfort from our lives, but to become skilled at feeling uncomfortable and moving anyway—and remembering that discomfort doesn't last forever! Again, this does not mean ignoring your sensations but opening to them, making space for them, as you move your body because you care about it.

In this chapter we'll be exploring more psychologically flexible and compassionate ways to embrace and overcome barriers like mental fatigue, chronic pain, low mood, and tiredness. Also, how to give up on trying to convince yourself to move, how to pace yourself when movement hurts, and how to use your heart to help you choose physical activity.

Reason 23: My job is not physical, so my body isn't tired after work, but my brain is so tired I just can't convince myself to move, despite knowing that if I go for even a short walk or move in some other way, I feel better and want to do more.

It's an uphill battle to try and convince a tired brain to do anything. The brain uses two systems to make decisions: a fast, intuitive, emotional system, and a slower, more deliberate, logical system. When you are fatigued, you're more likely to use the first, fast system, which leads you to follow your emotional impulse ("I'm too tired") more than your wiser, deliberate self ("Walking may help"). It sounds like your brain is fatigued from so much mental work, but counterintuitively, it's movement that may help revive it! Letting your mind wander along with your legs on a walk and getting blood flow to the brain is rejuvenating after all that mental work. Plus your body is probably screaming for movement after a long day of inactivity, which can be further stressing you out.

So, how can we get ourselves to go for a walk when our tired brain is running the show? First, stop trying to convince yourself. You are depleting even more of your mental energy by battling your exhausted brain. Throw in the towel in the battle with your mind and put your energy towards your heart and your feet.

Your heart knows what you care about, and your feet are going to get you where you need to go.

Get Out of Your Head and Into Your Heart

Imagine you could drop the decision to walk after work into your heart—not your head! What would your heart say about it? Why, in your heart, do you want to move more? If you had all the energy in the world after work, what would you really want to do? If your heart were in charge, not your head, what would it tell you at the end of the day? Write down at least one heart-based statement about walking in your notebook.

When you get home and your head says, "I'm too tired," listen to your heart instead. If it helps, you can put out a reminder for you to do this, like a picture or a note by your door. For example, I (Diana) have a sign above my front door written in calligraphy that says, *Enjoy walking.* My heart knows that walking is one of the most important aspects of my and my family's wellbeing. My heart wants me to walk when I can, to enjoy more of life. I keep the sign there as a reminder when I'm tired, my kids are protesting, my dog is being unruly, or I feel like I don't have enough time. Open up the door and enjoy walking!

Get Out of Your Head and Into Your Feet

Sometimes when we are tired it's best to bypass thinking altogether. Your head may be giving you a hard time, but your feet know what to do. You know this in other spaces. You get up and prepare for work even when your mind resists. You get out of bed to help your kids in the middle of the night, regardless of whether you feel like it or not. You're well-practiced in this approach already, you just haven't done with exercise...yet!

It's a powerful thing when you can learn how to override your mind with your action. Try this right now: Say "I cannot raise my hand" three times. Then, raise your hand as you say it. Could you do it? Great! That's an example of taking action that isn't fully reliant on conscious thought.

One way to support mind override is by turning your after-work walk into a habit. When a habit is formed, a part of your brain called the basal ganglia takes over, allowing your actions to become more automatic, reducing the need for conscious effort. The basal ganglia are also connected to your brain's reward system, so if you focus on the rewarding aspects of walking after work, it can further reinforce and strengthen the habit.

Make walking out the door a non-negotiable habit (go to pages 37–40 to learn more about habit formation): You come home (cue), put on your walking shoes and take the walk (behavior), then feel better because of it (reward). And you can make it even easier on yourself if you wear shoes to work that you can walk in anytime!

When you repeat the habit of walking after work, it will become more automatic over time and you'll also get in the habit of overriding your mind and acting with your feet. You may notice that your mind gets on board about ten minutes or so into the walk, which is a bonus, but not necessary. Your feet are running the show.

Rethinking Movement
Moving Before You're Too Tired To

The physical benefits to movement are there no matter what time of day you exercise, so the question becomes whether there is any benefit to experiencing them sooner in the day. Said another way, if exercise improves your mental clarity, attention span, and creativity, why not step into your worktime with all of these turned on? Not only can this help offset some of the mental fatigue you might be experiencing, it also solves the other problem of trying to fit in your first movement of the day at the end.

Mornings can be hectic—we can feel groggy to downright exhausted, there are breakfasts and lunches to prepare, work to finish, maybe kids to get out the door—but cultivating an early-morning movement habit could ultimately offer you more energy, setting the stage for a more dynamic day, making it easier to move all day long, including on work breaks and after work too. Not only do movement breaks help stop mental fatigue throughout the day, you're also saving yourself the energy costs of worrying about the fact that you haven't moved yet.

Reason 24: I have chronic pain from an illness. How can I approach moving more?

When you have medical complications such as an injury, chronic illness, or chronic pain, you might find that you flip-flop between stopping physical activity altogether and being overly ambitious and hurting yourself to the point where you are forced to stop.

Current research on pain management shows that both avoidance of activity and over-activity are linked to poorer outcomes like delayed healing, reduced mobility, and decreased pain tolerance. We need to aim for both/and here. Use *activity pacing* to make sure you aren't injuring yourself, and *activity stretching* to expand your comfort zone.

Activity Pacing

Activity pacing is an approach recommended in pain therapy that breaks tasks or activities into smaller bits so you can find a middle path between overdoing and under-doing. There are three main guidelines to keep in mind with activity pacing: Put your energy towards activities you value; base your activity amount on a pre-planned measure (e.g., minutes walking, reps of exercise, laps swimming); and gradually increase your activities based on a pre-planned quota.

Choose your valued activities. Make a list of the physical activities you engage in. Which ones do you value the most? Pick up to three most valued activities to try pacing with.

Define your baseline. Engage in your valued activity and record the time, distance, or number of times you can do it without having major medical complications/pain/exhaustion. Note that sometimes this process involves setting a baseline much lower than you expect. This is an important part of building up your tolerance; focus on what you can do, and don't worry about what you can't do right now.

Repeat your baseline activity for one week. Record your pain and any other complications on a pain-monitoring form. You may want to try the science-backed free online app SOMA developed at Brown University at somatheapp.com.

Increase by 10 percent. If you were walking for thirty minutes without serious complications, increase your walk to thirty-three minutes. If you were doing ten push-ups, try for eleven. (If your numbers are much lower than that, don't worry about it—just focus on the percentage of increase.)

Keep slowly increasing. Go slow to go far. If possible without experiencing worsening symptoms, increase by 10 percent each week. Build up the time on your tasks in a way that is sustainable.

Activity Stretching

As you pace yourself, also continue to challenge yourself in a sustainable way. Activity stretching is the act of gently moving to the edge of what our mind "thinks" we can do and expanding it. By moving outside your current comfort zone, you stretch it, making it bigger and thus making you more comfortable in a wider set of scenarios.

Be willing to feel tired while moving. You aren't going to feel your best every day. And you can still move your body, even when it's not at its best. By pacing yourself, you can slowly stretch and extend your comfort zone even when you are tired. Work on making that 10 percent increase, even when you're feeling tired.

Challenge your mind. Your mind is designed to give you advice to keep you safe, but sometimes your mind errs on the side of being overly protective. Challenge your mind's assumptions by acting independently from what your mind says.

Don't get stuck in a story. Our mind creates stories about ourselves to make sense of the world and predict the future. But when those stories define who we are and limit our range of possibilities, they box us in.

Without invalidating your true struggle, you can also zoom out and ask yourself...Are you sure? What is true and what am I adding on?

Things to Keep In Mind

Don't push your limits; stretch them. On a good day you may want to push yourself hard because it feels great. However, when you have a medical condition or chronic pain, slow and steady wins the race. Remind yourself it's not worth it to push yourself hard and then not be able to move for the next week! Stick to your pre-planned activity commitment.

Do small chunks frequently. If an hour-long walk worsens your symptoms, try distributing parts of your baseline activity throughout the day. Break the hour into six ten-minute walks.

Use one activity as a rest from another. One way to pace your moving is to alternate what you are doing. For example, rather than walking for twenty minutes and doing yoga for twenty minutes, try ten minutes of walking, ten minutes of yoga, then ten more of each. Sometimes the entire body doesn't need to rest, just certain parts.

If you have a flare-up, go back to your baseline and build up slowly again.

Finally, give yourself grace. Ability and disability are dynamic and change over time. Acknowledge the impermanent nature of your health. Caring for your body with pacing is caring for your health, even as it waxes and wanes.

Rethinking Movement
More on Ten Percent

Figuring out 10 percent of your baseline activity is simple when you're considering easily countable things like workout times, distances, and reps of an exercise, but how do you figure out how to practically add 10 percent of a yoga or spinning class? An activity-rich meetup with friends? What if you want to try something new and you have no baseline for that type of activity?

Start by thinking of every activity in terms of effort. No matter what the task, you can always find the overall intensity (i.e., how much effort the whole thing takes) and adjust it. You might not be able to keep the math perfect, but you can be a little qualitative in your approach and still honor the spirit of the 10 percent guideline. Maybe you want to try a new exercise video for lifting weights. Yes, you could just try doing just 10 percent of the video length to get your 10 percent—a six-minute movement session—but you might also be able to do a longer portion, or the entire thing, at 10 percent of your total intensity by, for example, keeping all the moves impact-free, taking small steps, and just trying the weightlifting motions without actually using weights.

If you're excited at the thought of joining in a live or online stationary cycling class for the dose of community, bumping music, and fun factor, you could attend just six minutes of class, or you could take it to 10 percent by ignoring all the instructor's intensity-building cues to increases resistance and jump in and out of your seat. Instead, pedal easily—beach-cruisin' effort!—throughout the full duration of class. You're still meeting the intention of the 10 percent rule in terms of pacing your energy, just in a different way.

I (Katy) have spent a lot of time in gym and exercise culture and I will say that it's absolutely common practice for people to come to a group workout, training session, or exercise video and do the session in a way that works for *their* body. Just check in with your instructor ahead of time when relevant—let them know that you're currently needing to manage your symptoms and will be staying "low and slow," and that you might also need to leave midway through. That's all totally fine; people who teach exercise are usually doing it because they love the way movement makes them feel and want other people to share in those same benefits. If you don't want to let your instructor know, that's also fine, just know that they might check on you during class if you're moving more slowly or resting more often because they are also monitoring everyone for signs of distress or overexertion.

If you've been passing on events like group hikes or family soccer, look for ways to get that 10 percent when you want to. Ask to be the goalie, where there's less running but you can still play with friends. Skip the hike around the park track, but show up later with a frisbee for some throws with friends. Take your swings in the softball game, but get a pinch-runner so you're fresh to hit in more innings later in the game.

When we talk about the 10 percent rule, it might feel small and discouraging—"I'm only able to work at 10 percent!" But that's not accurate. Adding 10 percent is working at your full capacity, when considering your capacity over a day or two. You're working at your 100 percent!

Reason 25: Menopause blues weigh me down and make me not want to do anything.

Just like going through puberty, the transition to menopause can feel chaotic and depressing and out of our control. It's also a lot of work to change the anatomy and physiology of our body—no wonder we're so tired. (And yet it seems we can't sleep. What's up with that?)

Approximately 80–90 percent of women who approach menopause report mild to severe physical or physiological complaints, with the most common being hot flashes, night sweats, vaginal dryness, depression, irritability, and sleep disorders. What's more, menopausal women have an increasingly sedentary lifestyle. As women age, their physical activity tends to decline significantly. About 29 percent of women aged 18 to 34 meet federal guidelines for aerobic and muscle-strengthening activities. However, this figure drops to 18 percent for women aged 50 to 64, and by the time they reach 65 or older, only 11 percent are meeting these guidelines.

Menopause, like puberty, is a normal and necessary stage of human development, and staying physically active can help a lot when it comes to managing the effects of this transition. Several studies have shown that being physically active improves menopause insomnia, hot flashes, and low mood. And engaging in resistance training plus aerobic exercise can protect muscle mass and decrease risk for heart disease. And yet, it's difficult to be motivated when we feel down. What to do?

In a qualitative study published in *BMC Women's Health*, researchers explored the key factors that played a role in perimenopausal and menopausal women aged forty to sixty-five being physically active. Three overarching themes emerged:

- **Daily routine:** Women were more likely to exercise when physical activity was part of their daily structure. E.g., "On Mondays, Wednesdays, and Thursdays I go to water aerobics."

- **Intrinsic motivation:** Women were more likely to engage in physical activity when they anticipated positive feelings with exercise. E.g., "I know I always feel good afterward."

- **Psychosocial support:** Women were more likely to engage in physical activity when it was linked to others. E.g., "Now I really can't bail, because everybody is expecting me."

Let's personalize these three factors.

Daily routine. How can you build movement into your daily routine? Be specific about the time of day, the days of week, and the cues that will remind you to move your body. Complete these prompts, and consider adding your new routine to your calendar.

Days of week I commit to exercise:

Time of day:

Type of moment:

Cues that will remind me to move:

Intrinsic motivation. What are the positive aspects of movement for you? How does it impact your mood, your energy levels, or your sleep? What do you look forward to when it comes to moving your body? Complete these prompts:

- Things I enjoy about moving as my body changes and ages:

- I look forward to moving as my body changes and ages because:

Psychosocial support. Who supports you in moving more? Who are the people you can move with? What classes or activities can you do socially? This can include online support groups and classes as well as in person.

- People/groups who support me in moving more:

- People/groups I want to move with:
- People/groups I can verbally share my commitment with:

By building in routine, intrinsic motivation, and psychosocial support, you will better be able to navigate the menopause blues with movement!

Rethinking Movement
Paring Down

The structure of the brain changes when we go through puberty and the brain changes again when we go through menopause. In both cases, this pruning away of unnecessary neurons is ultimately about efficiency. When we prune a tree, the removal of unnecessary parts is ultimately a pathway for the tree to flourish, and it's the same for the brain. Just as there is with tree pruning, there is a loss when we prune our brains (our transition away from childhood gets rid of all those unused neurons that would make learning a second or third language so much easier!), but we also end up with a brain best suited for our next biological phase.

According to Dr. Lisa Mosconi, neuroscientist, brain researcher, and author of *The Menopause Brain*, menopause is a renovation project on the brain that allows women to move on to a different, non-reproductive phase of life. Humans are one of the few animals gifted with time beyond their reproductive years, but that gift does come with this uncomfortable, rocky patch of transition that can feel like an emotional rollercoaster. It's like being a teenager all over again!

Imagine telling a bunch of moody teenagers all the reasons exercise would make them feel better. All Nike aside, saying "just do it" is not usually very effective with teens. Why would we expect something different from those navigating menopausal terrain? In both cases, there might be something more akin to deeper grief going on at the loss of the previous stage, and maybe even apprehension as to what's coming up. Why not lean into those bluesy feelings in an active way?

When I (Katy) was a teen, I used to walk my neighborhood, playing the Beach Boys' teenager anthem "In My Room" over and over again on my

Walkman. (For those youngsters out there, this took more than a tap on the "repeat" button; it required dedicating a full thirty seconds to rewind my cassette tape at the end of the song.) I walked the beach listening to heartbreak songs for hours at a time. And when I (Diana) was a teen, I'd stuff the top of my leotard and go to step aerobics classes with my mom and other forty-year-olds. I liked being around older women who seemed to have a few things figured out and were through the teenage angst. Now that I'm in perimenopause, one of my favorite things is to walk with seventy-year-old women who are on the other side.

What's your teenagery version of a more dynamic menopausal blues?

- Take a bath with lots of candles, then put on bluesy music while you do stretches in the dark.
- Blast speed metal while walloping a punching bag.
- Take a day off from talking to anyone while on a long hike or surf session.
- Meet up with your other menopausal peeps and have a bitching-about-it-while-biking session.
- Spend an hour at a batting cage.
- Find a wise older woman to walk and talk with.

Instead of looking at movement as a way to fix or turn off your feelings, you can look to your movement toolkit as a way to honor and move through your feelings.

Reason 26: I want to walk outside, but it's too cold.

The word that really catches my attention in what you're saying is *but*. You want to head out for a walk, *but* it's freezing outside. It feels like your mind is setting up a bit of a dilemma, like you have to pick one or the other. On one hand, you're eager to go for that walk; on the other hand, the cold weather isn't exactly inviting. Your mind is suggesting it's an either/or situation (check out page 54 for more on either/or thinking).

Building on the concept of shifting either/or thinking to both/and thinking, you can also change your *buts* into *ands*. This is a concept that ACT expert and researcher at Brown University Dr. Jason Lillis uses in his exercise interventions. By changing your *buts* into *ands*, you can make room for both of these thoughts to exist together. Let me show you what I mean by giving you some examples.

Instead of thinking, *I want to go for a walk BUT it's cold outside,* try *I want to go for a walk, AND it's cold outside.* Or you can adjust further: *I am excited about a walk, AND I'm aware of the chilly weather.*

See how this little shift in perspective can change things? It's not an either/or situation anymore, and suddenly, your motivation and outlook might start to shift too, as you look for solutions to a situation rather than give up in the face of an impossible obstacle.

Here are some other examples of changing *buts* into *ands*:

- I want to go for a swim, BUT I'm tired. → I want to go for a swim, AND I'm tired.
- I like how exercise feels, BUT it's hard to find time. → I like how exercise feels, AND it's hard to find time.
- I need to walk more for my back health, BUT it's uncomfortable to get started. → I need to walk more for my back health, AND it's uncomfortable to get started

- I want to take the stairs at work, BUT I'm pretty busy → I want to take the stairs at work, AND I'm pretty busy.

Change Your *Buts* Into *Ands*

Write a few of your *but* statements in a notebook and see if you can change them to *and* statements.

Notice that both can be present at the same time. One doesn't have to cancel the other out. When you replace *but* with *and*, you have a choice. You don't have to make the choice to move every time, and now you can see the choice.

Rethinking Movement
But, And, So...

Once you've changed your *buts* into *ands*, take this additional, practical step to help you get the movement you want: add a *so*. Not just the weakest Scrabble play ever, the word *so* is another way of saying *therefore*. The *so* after the *and* is a step that will help you get done what you wanted to do. Here are some examples:

I want to go for a walk, AND it's cold outside, **so...**

...I'm going to need an extra layer, mittens, and the right socks.

...I need to start uphill right away to get me nice and warm.

...I'm going to enjoy a hot bath when I get back.

I want to go for a swim, AND I'm tired, **so...**

...instead of doing an hour of laps, I'm going to go for twenty minutes and see how I feel, and get out if I need to.

...instead of doing a speedy swim workout, I'm going to see if a friend wants to join me in the pool to chat while using the kickboards.

...I'm going to lazily sidestroke and dog-paddle in the deep end while my kids show me all their dives and cannonballs.

I want to take the stairs at work, AND I'm pretty busy, **so...**

...when I hit my next lull in creativity and start scrolling mindlessly, I'll use this as a cue to go up and down the stairs once.

...I'll take seven minutes of my lunchtime to slowly walk the staircase.

...I'll ask a coworker to take the stairs with me so we can keep our discussion going.

By coming up with your *so...*, you're thinking through what you want long enough to come up with a mini-plan that cuts through some of the discomfort your mind was objecting to, and this can help make your wants—in this case for movement—happen. Don't forget to *so*, yo!

Reason 27: I'm grieving my dad, and feel like I'm carrying around a load of bricks. It's all so heavy and sad. I feel like I've lost my movement mojo.

Grief often feels like a heavy burden, making everyday life and activities seem like you are moving through molasses. It's entirely natural to feel a loss of motivation and energy during this time, as grief impacts your whole emotional and physical system.

Physical activity can help you move through the grieving process. Moving your body can give you a sense of freedom, offer a place to express your emotions, be a positive distraction, and enhance social support. Grief, especially in the early stages after losing a loved one, can also have a significant impact on your body. It often leads to heightened stress, affecting your body's cortisol levels, sleep patterns, and immune system, making it more vulnerable to getting sick. Grief can also trigger inflammatory responses, increase heart rate and blood pressure, and potentially lead to sleep disturbances. Physical activity can help keep your body healthy while grieving, counteracting some of this stress on your system.

Instead of seeing physical activity as something separate from the grieving process, let's consider some ways you can weave them together.

Create a Dynamic Movement Grief Ritual

Rituals can ground you, help establish a daily rhythm, and be especially helpful during times of stress and uncertainty. Unlike routines, which lack intentionality, rituals are meaningful practices that bring heart and purpose to what you are doing. Rituals don't have to be complicated or time-consuming, and they can be built into what you are already doing. I (Diana) have a client who has a grief ritual of walking around the public rose garden on Sundays and stopping to smell her mom's favorite roses.

Another client painted a rock with her dog's name on it and placed it by the road where they loved to walk together. When she heads out on the road she always brings a flower to place on the rock and is delighted to see that other dog lovers add to her little altar each week. How could you pair movement with a ritual that honors your loved one?

Remember Your Dad At His Best

When you have lost someone you love, it's a gift to them to remember them at their best. What physical activities did your dad love as a kid? What sports did he play? What type of exercise did he like as an adult? What physical activities did you enjoy together? Choose a few activities that remind you of your dad, and do them with him in mind. Your dad doesn't have the opportunity to move his body anymore, but you do. Move your body as a gift to him, celebrating the things he loved. You can even say, "This is for you, Dad" as you do it.

Grief walking

My (Katy's) dad was an avid exerciser, and his routine always included a daily walk. When visiting his resting place on the first anniversary of his death, my sister and I decided we would walk to the cemetery instead of driving. Yes, our trip took two hours instead of fifteen minutes, but we ended up connecting to him the entire time in a way that also connected us, joyfully, to our bodies and to his body, now gone. It felt so good! While it would still have been wonderful to only connect to him graveside, our walk *in memoriam* felt nourishing in an entirely different way. This walk's for you, Dad!

Rethinking Movement
Dynamic Grief

In her book *The Grieving Brain*, psychologist Dr. Mary-Frances O'Connor discusses how relationships make their way into our brain. The brain encodes a bond between our loved ones, and when they go, it's akin to phantom limb syndrome. Part of our own bodies—in our brains, where the overlap of you and a loved one exist—is now missing, and our brains have to update and change.

Although the grieving process is quite natural, it takes time and energy and also external support. Much like a splint or cast can aid in the natural process of bone or muscle-tear repair, we can choose daily practices that support healing.

Physical activity is helpful for many mental and physical health issues; bereavement can be hard on the body and is associated with physical and mental health concerns. So it makes sense to pair the two activities—grieving and exercising. But maybe you don't feel like "exercising off" the effects of grief for your own health when part of your life is missing. It's no wonder this approach might not be motivating.

Instead, think of ways physical activity can support your grieving process more directly. Look for therapists or grief support groups that offer dynamic options—e.g., walking therapy sessions. Wild Grief in Washington state is an organization that connects children, teens, and families to outdoor experiences (day hikes, backpacking trips, etc.) with other grieving peers. The Umbrella Project does something similar on the East Coast. Many places have walking or cycling groups just for those in the grieving process. Search for something similar in your area, or perhaps just ask if anyone in your weekly support group wants to meet up for a bike ride or hike to do some more processing.

While there's no doubt the physical benefits of being active are supportive, the loss of a loved one is also splinted by time in nature, with others, and embodied experiences that remind us that we are here, now, as we heal.

Reason 28: I'm on my feet all day as a hairstylist. The last thing I want to do at the end of my day is go for a walk. I just want to have my feet rubbed and watch a good show.

It sounds like some of the discomfort you're experiencing is physical (you've been using your body all day!) and some is psychological (you didn't exercise, so you feel like you need to add exercise but feel defeated because you can't). I (Katy) am here to give you your first movement reframe: **You're already getting lots of movement.**

Much of the discussion around needing to move more is general and directed to those with sedentary occupations. "Just move your body to break up so much sitting time." There is less messaging around the types of movement needed by those who already have physically active occupations. If it just takes "moving your body" to make our muscles and joints healthy, why do people in physically active jobs often experience joint pain and body fatigue—sometimes to the point of needing to quit their occupation?

For example, a review of forty-four studies examining musculoskeletal health of hairdressers showed that hairdressers give up their profession mainly for health reasons. Repetitive movements such as bending over the sink in an awkward position, the fine movements of holding and squeezing shears for hours, plus standing for prolonged periods of time can be hard on your body. So it's not just "getting enough" movement that we need. We have to make sure our overall movement diet is balanced.

And I (Diana) can give you a psychological reframe: It sounds like you are longing for some self-compassion! You had a long day, your body and mind are craving being cared for, and you give a lot of yourself to others (let me tell you—on the days I get a haircut, I have a bounce in my step all day! Thank you!). I wonder how you can build in some more kindness, understanding, and care for yourself throughout your day, and at the end of your day. Self-compassion is different from self-care and both may be important here.

Self-compassion is treating yourself with kindness, understanding, and acceptance during times of difficulty. Self-care is taking deliberate actions to care for your physical, emotional, and mental wellbeing. The primary difference is that self-compassion is more an internal practice, how you relate to yourself, and self-care is an external practice, how you demonstrate your care for yourself. Let's add both!

Self-Care Practices

First, your feet. Are there ways you can care for your feet while you work? Shoes that give your feet room to move? Mini stretches you can take while working? E.g., a calf stretch between clients, rolling your foot on a ball or frozen water bottle on your break?

Second, your mind. It sounds like you want to tune out during the end of your day. Hairdressers are about as close to therapists as you can get, and I (Diana) understand that! Is there a way to meet that need to tune out during the day, too? Take your mind for a wandering five-minute walk when a client is running late? Plug in your favorite music and tune out the world a bit while you clean your station? You mind is craving some downtime, and it deserves to get it throughout the day, not just at the end.

Self-Compassion Practices

Pay attention to your physical and emotional needs throughout the day. Ask yourself, what do I need here? Where am I hurting? Listen to your needs, and acknowledge them. Even if you can't give yourself what you need in the moment, you are caring for yourself and showing that your needs matter when you listen.

Notice how you are talking to yourself about your movement. Are you being self-critical? Setting unrealistic standards? What would you tell your coworkers if they were judging themselves in the same way? Can you offer the same kind advice to yourself?

Focus your mind on the parts of your work that you love to do. Sometimes the kindest thing we can do for ourselves is to shift our attention (remember the flashlight on pages 122–23!). Are there parts of your work that you enjoy, glean meaning from, or find psychologically rich? Amplify those parts, see if there are ways to do more of them, and when you are in them, be mindful and present with the positive experience. When you do this, you may feel less drained at the end of the day.

Rethinking Movement
Your Movement Diet

You movement diet consists of total movement (*movement calories*), larger categories of shape/efforts (*movement macronutrients*), and the smaller movements you make at all the different joints in your body. We balance a food diet by making sure we eat from a wide range of food groups and that the foods we pick also contain the minerals and vitamins we need, and it works the same for a movement diet. Our movements need to use a wide range of shapes and intensities, and be well-distributed throughout the body.

Like many occupations, hairstyling is active, but in a really repetitious way. Your hands, neck, shoulders, feet, legs, and lower back might be feeling exhausted from doing a lot of one movement over and over again. When it comes to the movement "food groups," you've got standing and fine-motor movements covered, but your heart and lungs haven't been fed. Your stepping, spinal-twisting, and sideways-bending muscles are starving.

It sounds like you're already tuning in to what movements your body needs when you get home. You're not wanting to be upright, because you've already done thousands of "being upright" reps. And guess what? Massage is a type of movement, and your instinct to get a foot rub at the end of the day is a good one; all the little muscles and tendons in your feet need a different type of movement to balance out a day of standing on them.

If you don't have a live-in body worker, rolling your feet on a tennis ball while watching your favorite show is a great way to get those movement micronutrients. And why stop at the feet? You know best the body parts that are aching; you can use a tennis ball or other massaging device to address any points of pain or tension.

Seated desk workers are advised to break up long bouts of repetitious sitting positioning with movement breaks, and active workers need similar advice. You need to infuse your hairstyling movements with some of that balance. You'll likely be bushed at the end of a workday because it's so active, so reserve fifteen minutes in the morning before work for some heart-and-lung-moving movement nutrients. Run up and down a staircase ten times, jump rope, have a low-impact dance party as you get ready for work. Pick three body-balancing stretches to do in between clients—bonus if they use the tools you've already got around. (Hold a broom horizontally behind you, palms facing forward, and slide your hands towards each other along the handle as much as you can to stretch your shoulders.) Change your shoes and give your feet and legs a rest *from standing* by taking them on a short walk at lunch.

When we build a nutritious food diet, we can pick the foods we like and that work for our bodies. Do you want vitamin C from an orange or a bell pepper? Do you want protein from a steak or beans and rice? Your body does need to be fed and watered certain movement nutrients, but you get to pick movements you like most or that work for your body best. You get to decide which ones make the cut, and then just roll with it.

5

I'm Stuck to My Screen!

These days it's hard to not feel bound to our devices. Computers, tablets, and smartphones have become the predominant way people in our culture are communicating. Texts with friends, parent-teacher communications, Zoom meetings for work, and top leisure-time activities like shows, movies, reading, and podcasts are all funneled through a digital highway.

There is no doubt that screentime is shaping our minds, bodies, and movement patterns. We feel addicted to our devices, we can see clearly that they're interfering with other things we need (and want!) to get done, and we aren't always sure what to do about it.

As you will read in the upcoming pages, many people feel "addicted" to their devices. We crave them when we don't have them in our hands, feel loss of control over our use, and sometimes continue using them despite adverse consequences. Most addictions are fostered by a rigid response to internal feelings (also known as psychological inflexibility). We use the addictive substance or behavior because it distracts or numbs us from things we don't want to feel or keeps around the good feelings we do want to feel. Maybe you scroll on your phone after work to avoid the same set of boring chores, even when doing them is part of the way you value being a responsible homeowner. Maybe you spend too much time editing your social feed and miss your morning exercise class because you were chasing likes. If you're using your phone to avoid discomfort or chase after pleasure, and it's going against your values, it doesn't matter whether you define yourself as "addicted" or not—it's time to reclaim your power.

Many of us are clearly correlating our devices and personal use patterns with problems in our lives (our movement habits, in this case), so we'll be addressing how to use psychological flexibility and your movement toolbox to address the phone that just won't leave your hand, time-sucking social media, and sedentary computer work. You'll learn how to structure your physical environment so that it supports movement no matter which devices you have around, how to use behavioral principles to create new tech and movement habits, and, of course, how to challenge inflexible assumptions that keep you thinking, *It's the phone OR exercise.* Spoiler alert: It can be both.

Reason 29: I struggle with tech addiction. It's hard to go for a walk when the alternative is much more dopaminergic—like Instagram, TikTok, YouTube, etc.

There's no debate that social media impacts your dopamine system and can be hard to stop using.

Platforms like Instagram, TikTok, and YouTube act a lot like addictive substances, triggering the release of dopamine into the reward pathway of your brain. But have you ever noticed that even though you want to do them, you don't always like the way it makes you feel? And that the things you want to do less in the moment (like walking) give you more satisfaction in the long run?

Why We Go Back for More

Our understanding of dopamine has evolved significantly over recent years. While it was once primarily viewed as the "feel-good" neurotransmitter responsible for pleasure, researchers now see it as driving craving and motivation more than direct pleasure. This is why we feel compelled to scroll on our phones even if it doesn't necessarily bring us joy. Dopamine makes us want to keep doing something, even if we don't really like it.

But that's not the full picture of why we become addicted. When your dopamine pathway is activated, your brain responds by downregulating dopamine production to maintain balance, or homeostasis. This means that after the initial surge, your dopamine levels temporarily drop below baseline, creating a feeling of discomfort or dissatisfaction. So, you click on another video to bring your dopamine up again. This cycle reinforces the behavior, driving us to keep going back for more and more, chasing the dopamine surge and avoiding feel the low feeling that comes when we stop.

Sure, dopamine is involved in the experience of pleasure, but other neurochemicals like endorphins and serotonin contribute more directly to feelings of contentment and liking something. So how can we get off this dopamine rollercoaster and do more of what we like versus what we want? By getting moving, of course!

The key here is to stop overstimulating your dopamine system and instead choose activities that balance out dopamine and other neuro-hormones. To do this you are going to need to learn how to ride out the urge to scroll and choose to move instead.

Primal tech

Our smartphones may also be capitalizing on our ancient brain's longing to move regularly. Throughout human evolutionary history, physical activity was an integral part of daily life. Hunter-gatherer societies, for example, had to be physically active to find and obtain food, build shelters, and perform other essential tasks for survival. Video games exploit our brain's longing to dig, throw, and jump, and the repetitive habit of scrolling and tapping on screens satisfies our ancient habits of repetitive motion.

Surf the Urge to Scroll

Urge surfing is a mindfulness tool used to help people with addictions cope with cravings without acting on them. Developed by smoking researcher Alan Marlatt, urge surfing involves staying present with your urge, noticing it rise and fall like a wave, without acting on it. You are like a surfer riding a wave—it grows, it peaks, and it comes back down again. No matter how big the wave of craving is, it will come back down. And the more you practice urge surfing, the better you get at it. You aren't fighting the urge, but rather noticing it, and allowing it to crest and fall. Here's how to do it:

1. Notice the urge. Next time you want to hop on Instagram or TikTok, choose to wait it out a little longer and surf the urge. Pay attention to the feeling of craving in your body. What does it feel like when you want to pick up your phone? What is the sensation of the urge like? Is it a rising feeling? A tingling feeling? A gnawing feeling? Where do you feel it in your body? Your chest? Belly? Head?

2. Stay with it. Ride out the urge, noticing it grow or get stronger. What happens to the sensation if you don't act on it? Watch it change like a wave.

3. Don't add a story. Stay with the pure level of sensation without adding a story to it like *this will never end* or *I can't handle this.* If you notice a story like that, go back to paying attention to the sensation in your body again and ride it, like a surfer on a wave.

4. Do some fancy tricks. Once you get better at urge surfing, you can practice surfing the urge while you choose an activity that is not related to the urge. For example, you can surf the urge to scroll—while standing on one foot and putting on your walking shoes. You can surf the urge to grab your phone—while doing squats with your favorite movement video. Sort of like a surfer doing fancy tricks on the board, no matter how big the wave is, you can move your body where you *want* it to go.

Want to Move More and Like to Move More

Sure, we can be motivated by our dopamine-craving system, but another reason we may want to do something isn't about dopamine hits; it's about values, and building a satisfying, worthwhile life. When it really comes down to it, what do you want deep down in your heart—to move or to scroll? Once you get the hang of surfing the urge, you can tap into this bigger want, i.e., your values. What brings you more contentment and long-term satisfaction?

Values help you want to move more. But they also help you *like* to move more too. Modern creations like junk food and social media make our brains less responsive to natural rewards like the sweetness of a carrot, the excitement of sprinting after a ball, or the satisfaction of digging in the garden. Where once a strawberry felt sweet enough, we now need strawberry Twizzlers to get that sweet feeling.

To get yourself able to like movement more, try being present with the pleasurable aspects that come with it. Pay attention to the difference between scrolling first thing in the morning versus the good feeling of getting outside and seeing the sunrise. Or the difference between rolling your neck on a break at work versus hanging your neck over a phone. These are small, and not the same big rush you get from Candy Crush, but the more you pay attention to them, the less you will like your phone, and the more you will like to move!

For movement to win out over phone use, you will need to surf the impulse to go to your phone right away, dig into your deeper motivation to move, and find the movements you like, savoring the subtle pleasure as you do.

Rethinking Movement
Walking Is Boring

When the choice is "fun times on my phone" or "going for a walk," you might need a different physical activity in order for movement to win out. If your social media apps feel more enticing than a walk, then a walk might not be the best mode of exercise for you right now. What are modes of physical activity you find more pleasurable, exciting, or stimulating, that you can set up against ninety minutes of Candy Crush? Playing ping-pong or tennis? Zooming around on a bike? Stretching on an aerial silk? Having a dance party? Taking a run with your friends?

When you do physical feel-good things like these, make sure to intentionally savor the good feelings—so that you help your brain notice how much you like moving. Be present in the positive experiences, amplifying them with your attention, to train your brain to want them more.

If you want to stick with walking because it's cheap and convenient, then you can also boost the "pow" in your walk by adding music. Once you're armed with the best playlist ever, see how that changes the way you feel about walking. Novelty is another way to give your regular routine a little "pleasure" boost. Do you take the same walk day after day? Change up your route. Add friends. Add a weighted backpack. Add a few intervals or running. Add a destination along the way. Or layer novelty *and* music by asking your friends, partner, or kids to make you a playlist that reveals itself once you're out on the move. Remember mixtapes and the excitement of waiting to hear what the next song would be? Talk about pleasing!

Another approach to increasing the excitement of your walk would be to meet yourself where you currently are—*both* having difficulty parting with your phone *and* wanting to move more—and pair your walk with your device in some way. Have you seen all the televisions atop the cardio equipment at the gym? People have been trying to take the attention away from workout efforts for decades. Like a mixtape, blending movement and tech is nothing new. You can gamify your workout with the help of smart device or physical activity app, and strive for a faster time or longer distance, track elements of your daily movement (steps, heart rate, etc.), or track your number of weekly workouts for digital rewards. Remember, the more you move, the more you'll downregulate your dopamine anyway, so using this aid in the short term can help you kick the addiction long term.

Reason 30: I think my top barrier to movement is my cellphone. Yesterday, after coming home from work, I thought to myself, "I'm going to relax with my phone for fifteen minutes, then go for a walk." That fifteen minutes lasted an hour and a half.

Our phones have become everything to us, even our relaxation devices! One thing to pay attention to here is, at what cost? And, is it really relaxing (and for how long)? Let's use psychological flexibility to find out.

What's the Cost?

One way to motivate us to change a behavior is to look at the short- and long-term consequences of what we are doing. Phone use can be like an invasive species, crowding out all other options. The phone is so quick, easy, and available, and it even comes with all those built-in "relaxation" apps. But at what cost? Pull out your notebook and answer these questions:

- How does using my phone to unwind after work affect my immediate state of relaxation and presence?

- If I continue to use my phone this way daily, what might the long-term impacts on my wellbeing and life priorities look like?

- What benefits do I feel I gain from this kind of phone-based relaxation?

- What experiences or practices could I be missing or "crowding out" by choosing to relax this way?

- What methods of relaxation resonate most with my core values and support the person I want to become?

Take an honest look at the short- and long-term consequences, and when you come home from work, bring those long-term consequences closer up. What life will you have missed out on if you do this every day? Practice perspective-taking and zoom out a bit on the time you're spending: If you were to add up 90 minutes of idle phone time every day for one year, that's 547.5 hours—almost 23 days.

Is that worth it to you? Now, if we were to add up 1.5 hours every day for twenty years, that's 456 days. More than a year of your life spent noodling on your phone after work!

Imagine all the relaxing, wonderful things you could do with that time instead.

What's the Point of Diminishing Returns?

You don't have to give up your "relaxation" phone time altogether, but it sounds like fifteen minutes was more what you were aiming for. One way to reduce your time on the phone is to stay present and pay attention to the point of diminishing returns. You know that point when another bite of cake doesn't taste as good as the previous one? There is a point of diminishing returns when it comes to phone use as well. When is the point where staying on your phone is no longer relaxing to you? When does staying on your phone actually make you feel worse? If you aren't used to checking in with yourself in this way, one way to do it is to set a time limit on your most-used apps (see details in the next section). When time's up, take a moment to notice what you are feeling in your body physically and emotionally. Do you notice you are getting less pleasure from what you are doing? That you are actually feeling more fatigued? Or maybe that you are feeling more anxious and agitated? These are all signs that you have hit a point of diminishing returns.

By paying attention to the point of diminishing returns, you can then choose to stop when you hit that point and try out some other relaxing activities with your body.

Off and Away

You also might need to set some digital boundaries. Willpower is no match for our phones, and part of taking committed action is setting up your environment to support your behavior change. You might want to try what schools are doing and practice what is called *Off and Away*. Make a list of places where and activities during which you'll turn your phone off and put it away in a drawer, bag, or another room. There are so many great opportunities to practice Off and Away:

- when hiking or walking with friends
- during an exercise class or video
- when you first get home from work
- when your kids walk into the room to greet you
- at mealtimes
- while watching a movie (ironically, phones can interfere with screen use! We have a strict "no two screens" policy in our house)
- when meditating, journaling, praying
- in work meetings
- while reading this book!

Then, utilize your phone's built-in screen-time features to help you limit your use. Mac, iOS, and Android all have screen-time functions that allow you to see how much time you spend on your phone and which apps you spend the most time on. You can then set these up to limit time on your phone. For example, using Apple's Screen Time or Google's Digital Wellbeing app, you can limit your screen time to fifteen minutes, and you'll get a signal once you've exceeded that. The only problem with this is that you can always ask for more time with a passcode. If you are so addicted that you usually overpower this block, give someone else your passcode so that only they open your phone.

Remember that the goal is not to eliminate phone use entirely, but to find a healthy balance that allows you to prioritize important activities like movement. You can gradually shift your habits by setting up environmental controls and paying attention to the point of diminishing returns when it comes to phone use.

Rethinking Movement
Relaxing (and Moving) with Your Phone

Our devices aren't only a barrier to movement, they can also be portals to moving more—we just need to set them up to be more supportive. If you find yourself on the phone and struggling with transitioning away from it, soften the transition by using your phone to get you moving by taking action ahead of time. Pre-load a few short (five or ten minutes long) movement videos to your phone or links to these classes on a memo. Choose one that's short and relaxing, one that's short and slightly more intense, and one that's a bit longer and moderately intense.

Next, find a spot for your fifteen-minute scrolling session (set the phone timer!) that can also double as a movement space. If you tend to nestle in bed or a big chair, opt to scroll lying on the floor in the living room—bonus points if you get your legs up the wall or do some spinal twists once you're down there. (Look, you're moving and scrolling at the same time!)

Before you start scrolling, open your five-minute video so it's ready, and set your intention—bonus points for saying it out loud—to do the video after scrolling. (In fact, you might want to just do it before scrolling to get it out of the way, but you don't have to.) After you've finished your scrolling time and then used your phone to give you a little movement segue in the form of a quick class, you're more likely to keep up the momentum and go for a walk. Or maybe just launch into the second short video, then take a walk. Or stay on the floor and just do the third video. No matter what you choose, at minimum you've brought the mountain to the movement, so to speak, which will make choosing movement, in any form, a little easier.

Reason 31: The first thing I do in the morning is go on my phone to check social media. I end up spending way too much time there and use up my precious morning walk time. It's annoying and I can't seem to break the habit.

Technology has the potential to intrude in every aspect of our lives if we allow it. Some strategies from the science of habit formation might help you reclaim your morning walk. As you learned on pages 37–40, most habits follow a similar pattern. Something cues you to do it, you engage in the behavior, and you are reinforced for doing it, so you do it again. Called a *habit loop,* the process looks like this:

Cue → behavior → reward.

In order to get yourself out on your morning walk, you need to deconstruct your existing habit of reaching for the phone following the steps below.

1. Identify your cues. Cues are the things inside and outside of you that trigger the behavior (grabbing your phone first thing in the morning). Are you picking up the phone to turn off the alarm? Do you fall asleep listening to music or podcasts on the phone, so it's already close to your hand? Does drinking your morning coffee cue up a scrolling session? Is the phone where you check messages from your kid's school, or the weather, or something else for work? Is there a game you like to play first thing?

   Once you know your triggers ahead of time, you are more likely to spot them and not go down the same mindless route. Once you've developed your cue-awareness, you can either change your environment to reduce those cues (e.g., get a digital clock for your nightstand so you don't need to use your phone as an alarm clock), or to replace the behavior with a more values-aligned one (e.g., when you wake up in the morning and grab your phone, take it with you on a walk).

2. Structure your environment to support new behavior. One of the best ways to change a habit is to change your environment. In your case, there are two ways you can change your environment.

   • Increase phone friction: Make it harder to do the behavior you don't want to do. Consider introducing some obstacles to make your phone less convenient. Charge it in a different room, eliminate the most addictive apps from your phone, or configure your phone so that it's not accessible until after a specific time of day.

   • Decrease exercise friction: Remove as many barriers to morning exercise as possible. For example, you may want to sleep in your exercise clothes, take your coffee with you while you walk, or keep your yoga mat out on the floor by your bed.

3. Reward physical activity. Make sure to reward yourself for choosing to go out for a walk instead of reaching for the phone. You can even use your phone to help with this! You can use your phone as a reward tool—you can have that scroll session or play Wordle after you take your walk. Or you can gamify your workout using an exercise app that incorporates tracking features, interactive games, or "complete the circle" technology to make your exercise routine more engaging and rewarding.

   You have the power to create a new habit loop first thing

in the morning. Using the techniques above, your new habit might look something like this:

Cue: wake up and turn off my digital alarm clock →
Behavior: go for a walk → Reward: check Instagram as soon as I get back!

Rethinking Movement
Set Your Alarm

The difference between something being a tool and a weapon often boils down to how you use it. It seems like everyone was given a phone with all its massive potential without any sort of direction as to how to wield it in a way that's supportive, not destructive, to your biology. When you can't put it down, at least put it to work in a better way.

For decades, folks have been advised to schedule their workouts on their calendar, because doing so helps you not only remember that class or walk you wanted to take, but it's a gesture that serves to remind us that physical activity is just as important as any other task we need to get done in a day. A modern twist on this old advice is "set an alarm for your morning walk." If you've set an alarm to wake you up, why not set an alarm on your phone that goes off twenty minutes later (maybe right in the middle of your scrolling)? Why not label that alarm with a note that also pops up on the screen: MORNING WALK REMINDER! YOU WANT THIS! I LOVE YOU! Then take your own advice (and your phone, if you must) and get that dose of morning movement you yourself call precious.

Reason 32: I work at a computer all day. I am a grinder. And though I know I'm too sedentary and I try to move a bit every hour, taking time for movement often feels like an indulgence that runs counter to my creativity and productivity at work. If things are flowing, I hate to break that up, and then at the end of the day I realize I've hardly moved at all.

Sometimes we feel like movement competes with other things we value, like work performance. It sounds like you care a lot about your work, love being in flow, and fear that getting up to move will interfere with your productivity. It also sounds like your identities of being a "grinder" and a "mover" come into conflict. Which do you choose?

There are two assumptions that you may want to get more flexible with:

1. Moving at work makes you less productive.
2. To be a grinder, you can't be a mover.

Let's use cognitive flexibility and perspective-taking to find some mental wiggle room so you can be both, and so much more!

Moving Makes You More Productive, Not Less

There's a large and growing body of research showing that exercise and movement improve your mental performance. Specifically, moving your body increases creativity, attention, cognition, and mood—all things that will make your grinder-self grind even better! For example, when research participants took a test while walking, their performance on a creativity task increased by 81 percent compared to taking the test while seated. And if you can add some movement into your work, you may actually be more efficient at it. In small study where radiologists read CT scans for lung cancer while seated or at a walking desk, they were equally accurate in detecting lung nodes but were quicker to finish their assessments when walking.

Moving your body also builds a better brain. Experimental and clinical studies have shown that exercise increases gray matter in your frontal and hippocampal regions (areas of your brain involved in memory and attention), increases neurotropic factors (which are like fertilizer for your neurons), and increases blood flow (which supports brain activity).

Exercise boosts concentration and focus, helping you sustain your attention on tasks that require mental effort. And acute bouts of vigorous movement have been shown to lead to higher positive emotions and energetic feelings that last for hours. Not only do you have more positive emotions, you are better at regulating negative ones when you move your body.

Given all of that, dear grinder, why don't you test it out for yourself—prove your mind wrong, and see that you can be an even better grinder when you fit in the movement. Try adding some short movement breaks throughout your day, or move while you work (see some ideas for how to do this below) and assess for yourself. Does adding movement into your workday improve your mental performance? How does it impact your creativity? Your focus? Your emotion regulation? In other words, does moving more improve your work performance?

Grind It Out

The next thing to get more flexible around is your identity as a grinder. When we rigidly hold identities like "I am a grinder," "I am a high achiever," or "I am a perfectionist," we can box ourselves into one role and fail to see our complex human selves. Are there other identities you hold in the workplace besides "grinder"? When you hold tight to the identity of being a grinder, does it get in the way of your values, or lead you to get down on yourself when you don't measure up to whatever a "grinder" means? Let's unpack this a bit more with perspective-taking.

Imagine it's the last day of your career, you're about to retire, and your colleagues have gathered to toast and roast you, sending you off to happy travels. How would you want them to describe you? You can include *grinder* on that list, but also include other qualities. What values did you bring to the workplace? How do you want to be remembered? What do you want them to say about how you took care of yourself? And how do you want to feel physically and energetically as you get ready to launch into your golden years? Will you be burned out or refreshed and ready to travel the world?

Get out your notebook and write down your retirement toast. After you write it down, underline the parts that highlight your values. How can you live out those values now, as you grind away at work? You are more than a grinder; that's just one of many roles that make up the complex human that you are, and there are a lot of ways you can grind while living out your other values.

A note on grinders

It's not uncommon to use grinding (at work, in sport, in the garden) to avoid feeling things like grief, anxiety, and sadness. When we use busyness to avoid those feelings, guess what? Other feelings can be blocked as well, including those communicating our body's need to move.

Grinders, try taking a pause a few times a day and allow any blocked, uncomfortable feelings to show up. Use your acceptance skills to make room for them and listen. Is there anything they are telling you that point to your values? Act from there.

Rethinking Movement
When You Are (and Are Not) in the Zone

Dear grinder, not all movement requires taking a break from being productive; there are a lot of ways you can keep your body moving while your mind stays busy working on a computer. Depending on your body and office-etiquette needs, you could use a standing desk, walking pad, or wobble board underfoot, all of which offer some amount of movement. Opting to call instead of emailing (so you can potentially be standing, stretching, or even walking) is another way to stack productivity with movement while also getting work done.

Don't forget your breaks. Lunch and other breaks you might be fortunate to have are great places to fit in smaller "movement snacks" that not only break up longer bouts of sitting, but also positively impact focus, creativity, and productivity.

That all being said, we can also appreciate not wanting to disrupt your flow state. From one grinder to another, I (Katy) have found there are certain types of work I can only get done with sustained "in place" time that I don't want to interrupt with a movement break.* However, I rarely stumble into this zone unknowingly. I know when a flow state is likely going to happen for me, because it typically takes a clear intention ("I'm going to write Chapter 5 today!") and a long period of uninterrupted time (which I need to schedule in advance). So if flow state is your best way of working, you don't actually need to interrupt it. You just need to take an honest look at your daily work calendar and notice when breaks are naturally going to occur already in the day—around meetings, shifts in tasks, lunch, etc.—and use those as cues for a quick stand-and-stretch, mini-walk, or position change. Identify any other cues that remind you you're not in a flow state. Leaving your current "big project" to frequently check your email or send non-urgent messages on software like Slack is, according to Cal Newport, author of *Slow Productivity*, a sign of "pseudo-productivity"—you're expending a good deal of effort, hoping to make progress, by doing a lot of unnecessary work-*like* activity. Yes, you are definitely at work and staying busy, but you're not really in a "deep work" state.

Other cues that you're still on the computer but no longer grinding: visiting non-work-related websites, or making those social media laps (frequent, routine, usually brief check-ins on your social media sites of choice). Your mind is trying to take a break by "stepping away" from work; take that as a great cue for logging some actual steps (or bends, or twists), not only for the body benefits but as a form of mental rest. Once you learn to recognize when you're in the flow and when you're not, use the "not" signs to cue you to grind out those movement breaks instead.

*When I do a thorough self-check-in and look hard at my calendar and see a deep work session coming up the next day, I choose to get early-morning movement to support the day's flow state, and I also set my workspace up so I can stand, wiggle, and fidget my body while my mind is otherwise occupied in place.

6

My Environment Makes It Impossible!

Some barriers to movement are truly external and not always fully addressable through behavior change or psychological means alone. Our context matters when it comes to movement. When we don't have safe places to move, when we lack finances to pay for childcare or a gym membership, or when the environment is not supportive in terms of weather or air pollution, it can be extra difficult to figure out how to get the movement our body needs.

Social determinants of health, such as access to health care, a safe neighborhood, job security, clean air, and access to education, have a huge impact on our physical activity and health.

Social determinants of health also contribute to inequalities in health outcomes. Populations that may be more susceptible to health disparities include communities with low income, people of color, those who are unhoused, pregnant women, and children. Environmental factors such as noise pollution, air pollution, lack of green space, and climate change are also likely to impact our ability to move our bodies outdoors. People who don't have a safe area to go to are less likely to exercise, which raises their risk of health conditions like obesity, diabetes, and heart disease. Environmental factors also disproportionately impact communities of color and low-income populations.

Still, there can be creative, flexible responses to these external environmental barriers that make it easier to deal with them or at least move around them, and that's where we can help. In addition to offering the same psychological tools and movement reframes, this section also includes ways you, concerned citizen, can take larger-than-yourself action when it comes to many of society's systemic problems that ultimately impact all of our movement (and beyond).

Systemic, larger-than-ourselves barriers can create feelings akin to grief. We all expect a safe place to walk, clean air to breathe, and enough time and money to take basic care of ourselves, and when we don't have these things, we feel a loss. We must create space to process and grieve these losses, and also figure out how to move forward despite them.

You deserve to be free to move—even in difficult contexts. In the solutions ahead we'll be covering: advocating for, and creating, safe spaces to move; identifying how your mind gets in the way of creative solutions; and how to use mindfulness and acceptance to increase your resilience and commitment to action, advocacy, and allyship.

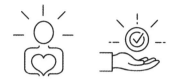

Reason 33: I have a lack of safety in my immediate area and a lack of resources to get to "nature." It's hard to go for a walk in an unsafe neighborhood, and I don't have the means to go to safer areas.

Before we offer strategies for staying active in an area where you feel unsafe, it's important to pause and acknowledge the difficult emotions that come up around this. You might feel anger, sadness, frustration, or fear. It's natural to feel a sense of injustice here. After all, everyone deserves the freedom to walk in their neighborhood without fearing for their safety. Recognizing and validating these emotions is a powerful first step. Practice acceptance—acknowledge that while these feelings are uncomfortable, they are valid responses to your circumstances. They tell you what you care about—which in this case may be your right to feel safe moving your body.

Create Your Own Pockets of Safety

When you feel unsafe, it can send your body into high alert. This chronic activation of your threat system is draining, and it's not good for our body or our mental health to feel stressed all the time. By creating pockets of safety, you can build a sense of centeredness and security within yourself. Once you build this safety inside, you can carry it with you wherever you go. When your alert system needs to turn on, it can do its job, and then you can return to your centered home base. Here are a few ideas for how to do this with self-compassion.

Create an inner safe space. Start by tuning in to your breath. In moments of tension, slowing your breath and focusing on a longer exhale can cue your body to relax, sending a signal to your nervous system that it's okay and safe. Sometimes, simply pressing your feet into the ground and feeling the solid support beneath you can offer a reassuring sense of connection and stability. You might also find it helpful to focus on a point of stillness within your body—perhaps placing a hand over your heart or belly—and letting your attention rest there, reminding yourself that you can always return to this centered place inside.

As part of this inner safety, try speaking to yourself in a way that feels reassuring and kind. Compassionate self-talk might include simple phrases like "I am here for you," or "Just this moment, I am safe," or "I've got you." Speaking to yourself with kindness builds a sense of inner refuge you can turn to anytime.

Build a mental safety map. Consider creating a safety map in your mind by imagining familiar places in your area that do feel more secure—local stores you could pop into, the homes of people you know you could knock on, or well-lit public areas. Visualizing these safe spots helps remind you that while there are areas that feel—or are—less safe where you live, there are also places where you can feel protected. There are always good people and safe places around us, even in the most challenging spaces. Having this mental map offers a sense of choice and control.

Create physical safety pockets. There are also practical ways to increase feelings of safety while walking. You might invite someone to join you occasionally, as walking with a friend or group can be physically safer than walking alone. Some people prefer to walk without headphones to stay aware, while others find that listening to an uplifting podcast or soothing music helps bring more peace of mind. Find what feels right for you. Letting someone know your route and expected return time is another way to create a layer of security around your routine. These small acts of precaution and connection can help build confidence as you move through your environment.

Making change

It's not up to any individual to eliminate systemic barriers to movement. Advocacy and policy changes are needed at the level of public health organizations, educational systems, transportation, and housing to address people's living conditions. Still, there are ways we can take personal action towards systemic change.

Contacting your representative is a great way to get started. Call, email, or write a letter to your local representative and let them know that creating safe places to walk in your neighborhood is an important issue for you as a voter. Get informed on propositions that support municipal improvements such as sidewalks, lighting, traffic calming, parks, and greenways. Here's a sample letter you can send that includes your name, the fact that you live in their district, and what you would like them to vote for or against.

Hi, my name is (YOUR NAME HERE). My zip code is (YOUR ZIP CODE HERE). As your constituent, I would like you to vote for the recently proposed measure that will require the department of transportation to add sidewalks and lighting for safety when planning major paving projects. I support all forms of improvements that create safer and greener spaces for our community to walk outdoors. If you vote for legislation that negatively impacts our access to physical activity, I will be voting against you in the next election.

Rethinking Movement
Finding a Safe Area to Move

After lack of motivation and lack of time, lack of adequate space for movement is a top barrier to moving more.

When you're living in an area that's unsafe for walking, that doesn't mean all movements are off the table for you. You can put your attention towards the movements you can do inside your home, or a garage or yard if you have one. This can be as simple as setting an exercise mat near a television (there are exercise videos and YouTube routines for just about any type of movement you'd like to explore from the comfort of your own safe space) to something larger: a walking pad or treadmill, a few hand weights and a small wall mirror to check your form, a jump rope, etc. Gyms and other indoor movement spaces are also options.

For the times you want to get outside and walk—especially if walking outside is your jam and you don't want to swap it for other types of movement—start keeping a pair of walking shoes with you, so you're ready to take advantage of the times you're already in more walkable areas: around your place of work, before and after school drop off, when visiting friends, grocery shopping, etc. This won't take more total time, you're just distributing the same "neighborhood walking time" to different parts of your day, but you'll definitely need to plan ahead the first few times until you establish a new pattern of when and where you're getting your walking done.

Reason 34: Exercise costs too much.

Finances can be a very real barrier to movement. Data from the CDC show that people who have less money are less likely to exercise. The percentage of adults who meet guidelines for both aerobic and muscle-strengthening activities decreases as family income decreases. Availability of free time, access to safe places to move, childcare, and the cost of gym memberships can all be barriers to moving your body if finances are tight.

Even with the reality of financial constraints, there are some things under our control when it comes to movement, like our perspective and our action.

Shift Your Perspective

Even if there are external reasons to blame, be careful not to get stuck in a helpless, negative self-story about why you can't move. Remember, self-stories are beliefs we hold about ourselves and the world around us that shape our perception and actions. When you get stuck in a self-story like "I can't exercise because it costs too much," you might be falling into common thinking traps like:

- The confirmation bias: You seek evidence to confirm your belief that exercise costs too much and ignore evidence that contradicts your view. (See some evidence in the "Rethinking Movement" section below and see if that shifts your thoughts on the matter!)

- The authority bias: You place greater importance and weight on the opinions of people in authority and don't take a closer or deeper look for yourself. For example, you buy into

messaging from fitness experts or companies that suggest
you need expensive classes, equipment, or outfits to exercise.

- The anchoring effect bias: Your decision-making is influenced by an "anchor"—a piece of information you once
  received that you rely upon too heavily when making
  decisions. For example, your anchors could be that your
  friend told you her yoga class cost thirty dollars, or that you
  read an article about exercise being out of reach for many
  due to the cost, and since then you've decided that all forms
  of exercise are too costly for you.

Catch yourself when you are caught in these limiting perspectives, and
ask yourself, what is under my control? Where can I make active choices
that align with my goals and values, even when finances are tight?

Rethinking Movement
Take Action with No-Cost Movement

There is no doubt that there are some pricey pathways to exercise. And
there are also a great number of ways you can get exercise for free, and
it's all the same when it comes to mind and body benefits. Here are some
ideas to consider:

- walking
- running
- rucking
- dancing
- bodyweight exercises/calisthenics
- pretty much any type of exercise class (hundreds, if not
  thousands of options—including varying length and skill
  level—on YouTube)
- exercise videos from the library
- swimming (lakes, ocean)

- chin-up bars/exercise circuits in local parks
- pick-up games: soccer, basketball, ultimate frisbee, etc.
- libraries often have free bus and entry passes to get to nearby state and national parks as well as other outdoor gear like backpacks, sleds, and even kayaks available to check out.

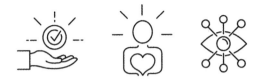

Reason 35: Outdoor air quality is impacting my ability to move. Last week my family was cooped up inside for over three days because of the wildfire smoke. And today there's an ozone alert (though we got some walking in before it started). I did bring a jump rope inside and we try to do other movements, but not being able to walk outside is a HUGE bummer.

There are plenty of places in the world where there are almost always dangerous levels of air pollution. The climate is shifting, and we are feeling its impact on all aspects of living, including physical activity levels. In many communities the impact is palpable: Unsafe beach conditions, extended periods of water conservation, hurricanes, flooding, excessive heat, fire evacuations, and debris flow during storms are a new normal. It doesn't seem like anywhere is unaffected.

Take a Metta Moment

This is a great place to connect to the reality that many people around the world are in this situation—and have been for a lot longer than us, whether because of natural phenomena or human pollution. We can acknowledge our eco-grief and offer compassion not only to ourselves, but also for the people, plants, and animals that are impacted by pollution, habitat destruction, and climate change. Compassion can flow in multiple ways here, and sometimes offering compassion to others who are struggling makes you feel less alone and helps you feel our common humanity—no one is immune from climate change and environmental damage, although some people are more impacted than others.

The word *compassion* comes from the Latin word *compatio*, which means to "suffer with," and compassion comes with the motivation to do something about it. One thing you can do is open your heart and aperture to a larger view than just you and your family. Think about all the beings impacted by poor air quality, and offer them some *metta,* or words of loving kindness. Here is a phrase that I (Diana) was given when I was facing loss, that I find particularly helpful.

Start with giving yourself some loving kindness:

> May I be one with myself
>
> May I be free from suffering
>
> May I experience peace of mind and in body

Then consider the families, children, animals, and ecosystems that are experiencing climate distress and send them loving kindness:

> May we be one with each other
>
> May you be free from suffering
>
> May you experience peace of mind and in body

When we activate compassion, we feel less alone, connect to our larger system, and shift our mindset from "this is only happening to me." This mindset shift can also help us take the next step, which involves accepting reality so we can take action.

Accept Reality and Shift Your Mindset

Christiana Figueres, coauthor of *The Future We Choose* and a key figure in global climate strategy, emphasizes the need to *both* acknowledge our grief over climate change *and* move from a mindset of helplessness to empowerment (for more on both/and thinking go to page 55). Figueres advocates for three key mindsets:

Stubborn optimism. Stubborn optimism transcends mere hope; it's about actively shaping a sustainable future for our planet through deliberate actions. You already are taking deliberate actions towards stubborn optimism by getting outside when you can, and bringing movement inside when you can't. How else can you use your body to bring the future you want closer? Embrace being a stubborn optimist!

Radical regeneration. Our planet possesses a remarkable ability to regenerate, and your physical activities can support this regeneration. Consider how you might use your own energy as a renewable resource to lessen the burden on Earth. For instance, could you choose walking or cycling over driving on clear days? Opt for less driving during smoggy conditions? Replace leaf blowers with brooms and rakes? Carry dishwater outside for your plants? Perhaps even grow some of your own food?

Endless abundance. Our planet is rich with renewable resources: the sun's energy, wind's power, and water's force. Similarly, you possess renewable personal resources—your values, your attention, and your action. Values like compassion, love, and creativity endlessly regenerate, offering unlimited potential for positive impact. Reflect on how these values can shape your approach to climate change. Ask yourself: How can my family and I channel our values to favor renewable resources over fossil fuels? Shifting your attention to what is beautiful, alive, and healthy right here and now can boost your mood and remind you that even in the smokiest of days there are things to savor, including physical activity (see below for some ideas). And shifting your action to where you have agency can renew your motivation to move.

Rethinking Movement
Seasonal Exercise Shifts

If you want to stay physically active throughout life, you need to be able to adapt your movement plan to your current age and stage. We will all experience times in our lives where things change, sometimes abruptly. Disease, injuries, divorces, and yes, even environmental disasters can all affect our movement options. The one constant in life is that everything changes, and there's often very little we can do to control things outside of our sphere of influence.

Being physically and psychologically resilient in the face of change takes flexibility—the ability to not hit an obstacle like a brick wall and instead move around it like water. Now, water is still having to change its course—it's not getting through without having to bend, pivot, and some-times bubble over with effort—but you can imagine that a stiff substance, like an ice river, would have much more trouble with the task. Changing course is much less of a jolt when you stay flexible.

When it comes to wildfire season, flexible movement plans might look like taking full advantage of any smoke-free days or periods of the day, and having your seasonal indoor movement plans ready ahead of time. Get a short-term pass for the local indoor pool and make daily swims/water play the season's movement macronutrient. Check in with indoor gymnasiums (try churches, schools, and recreational facilities) about your plan to bring a big group of people (don't forget the kids!) for a couple of hours of outdoor games (tag, ball, capture the flag, drum stalking) to play inside. At this point, a wildfire season is no longer sneaking up on us, and being ready with a movement plan that works can decrease your feelings of helplessness over the movement portion of the situation.

And keep your movement connected to your values: Are there things you might be able to do in other parts of the year—physically active things—that can positively impact wildfire season? Are there volunteer brush cleanups in your neighborhood or public lands to participate in? Does anyone need help rebuilding?

We can shift our moves seasonally (most of us do already; some of us just have to add "smoke season" to our calendar), and we can also shift how we move all year so our communities can thrive through these changing seasons.

Shifting your mindset, cultivating a sense that you are not alone, and moving more seasonally can help you carry the load of emotions surround-ing climate change. Many others share feelings of dread, anxiety, and grief. Explore platforms and communities where you can connect with others who share these feelings. Together, you can foster the courage, acceptance, and stubborn optimism needed to keep moving as our climate changes.

- Looking for an ongoing, structured group to process your emotions about climate change? Check out goodgriefnetwork.org

- Want to share your feelings with others but don't have a lot of time or don't want an ongoing commitment? Climate Awakening offers small group sharing sessions online. climateawakening.org

- Want to host your own climate circle in person or online? The All We Can Save Project offers you a step-by-step session guide. allwecansave.earth/session-1

Reason 36: The car dependency that has been created in North America over the last seventy-five to a hundred years has absolutely crushed the ability for many people to get outside and move as part of their daily living. It's too unsafe to walk or to bike anywhere.

Car dependency can be a real drag—especially if you want to get places by biking and walking and there is no real safe way to do it. It's frustrating when there are no bike lanes, you're walking next to a lot of exhaust or car noise, and there's no sidewalk to get where you want to go. This car-centric lifestyle has also shaped our daily routines, crowding out body-powered transportation.

But that doesn't mean it's *always* unsafe to walk or bike places where there are cars. Sometimes we experience something as very unpleasant and interpret it as unsafe. In psychology this is called *emotional reasoning*. Emotional reasoning happens when we believe that what we are feeling reflects reality, regardless of the evidence or facts. For example, if you fear biking or walking around cars, you might believe that it is unsafe. Or if you feel like cars have crushed our ability to go outside, you may believe that is true for most people. So how can you tell if something is emotional reasoning, or a fact? You have to look into it a bit more! Are there places where cars and movers safely co-exist? There are a lot!

In Boulder, Colorado, where I (Diana) went to graduate school, bike lanes are plentiful, and even on the coldest mountain days you'll see students and faculty beating out the traffic, pedaling uphill. And despite the car dependency in Southern California, more and more towns there are blocking off main shopping areas for pedestrians only, adding bike lanes, and creating bike-sharing programs. At UCLA (another college campus) it's wild and wonderful to see how many people are zipping around on skateboards and bikes! Many big US cities, like Baltimore, Cleveland, and Chicago, are actually known for high walkability scores, and there's been a surge of revamping the markings and routes of bike and walking paths in other places too.

While our emotions can skew the facts, they also can point us to what we care most about. If you are angry or afraid that cars are replacing physical transportation, there are values driving those strong emotions. What are they? Why do you care so much? Is it because you value keeping our air clean? Cultivating social connection? Taking care of public health? Preserving the sound of nature? Or something else? To take action on that value, I would recommend creating some values-based SMART goals around physical activity and car culture.

Set a Values-Based SMART Goal

A SMART goal is:

Specific: What specific action can you commit to that reduces your car dependency while also getting you moving? How will this support your value?

Measurable: How will you measure whether you are successful at reaching your goal (e.g., you could measure miles walked, biked, or skateboarded vs. miles driven)?

Achievable: Set a goal within your reach. Don't aim so high that you can't follow through. For example, think about yourself on your most tired, unmotivated, or rushed day, and then set a goal you could meet even then.

Relevant: Make your goal relate to your life. Remind yourself of your values and why you are making this change.

Time bound: When will you carry out this action? How long will you do it for? When will you check back in to assess if you are successful?

Your commitment to moving more signifies your dedication to your values, even when faced with challenges. When you get discouraged, remember that just because you feel a certain way, it doesn't mean your feeling is always true, and you can be part of the exception when it comes to the trend towards car dependency.

Rethinking Movement
Log Some Steps on a Walk Audit

While car culture is definitely dominant in many places, there are also many city departments and organizations working not only on ways to support safe, human-powered transportation, but on mobility justice too—the ability for everyone to freely and safely walk or roll through public spaces, regardless of identity.

One of the first steps taken to assess the walkability of an area is a walk audit. During a walk audit, an individual or group moves through a specific area or route looking at who is using this path and why, the markings and signage at street crossings, the amount of traffic, the state of the sidewalks, and the general street safety. Once completed, the results can be shared with neighborhood groups, school PTOs, elected officials, and other community leaders.

Walk audits are not only a good way to discover local areas that are safe for walking, rolling, or biking; they're also a great way to stack your personal movement needs with community service. Consider starting a regular walking group that explores new areas of your town or city every week while also auditing. Going with a group of people of different ages and stages might also reveal elements of walkability you hadn't thought of before. What's it like crossing the street when you move at a slower pace? How would someone in a wheelchair navigate this area without sidewalks? Are there places to use the bathroom, or benches to sit and rest? Is there a bus stop but no place to cross the highway safely?

Walk audits are also great to do with kids. They get kids moving outside and also thinking about city design and civic responsibility.

I (Katy) actively support my values around walkability by participating in walk audits, supporting larger political organizations like America Walks, and simply walking in as wide a variety of places as I can. Yes, there are cars everywhere, but there are also a lot of places to walk when you look closely. There aren't nearly the number of people lobbying for active transportation as there are lobbyists for cars and public transportation, and there are more cycling lobbyists than walkers. So, do the work and take the walk when you can. Download a Walk Audit Tool Kit from AARP (aarp. org/livable-communities/getting-around/aarp-walk-audit-tool-kit.html).

Reason 37: As a person of color, I fear I will be profiled if I run early in the morning or in the evening at my local park. It's my favorite place to jog, and it becomes dangerous and stressful for me because I don't feel safe.

It's maddening that you can't jog in your favorite place. And it makes complete sense that you fear you will be profiled, as racial profiling is a serious issue that discourages people of color from engaging in positive health behaviors like outdoor exercise, especially in predominantly white spaces. This is extra concerning because racial discrimination has negative effects on physical health and health disparities, and there's a disproportionate prevalence of obesity, diabetes, and cardiovascular risk in communities of color. And all of these conditions are improved with physical activity.

If you are feeling hypervigilance, dread, or anxiety about exercising in white spaces, your feelings are substantiated. According to data presented on the ACLU website, 41 percent of Black Americans say they have been stopped or detained by police because of race, and 21 percent of Black adults report being victimized by police. The danger for people of color exercising in white spaces was confirmed horrifically when Ahmaud Arbery, a twenty-five-year-old Black man, was brutally murdered while he was jogging in his predominantly white neighborhood.

In a paper titled "Running While Black" published in the journal *Preventive Medicine Reports*, Lyndsey Hornbuckle writes, "While attempting to overcome any barrier to a health behavior change can be difficult, battling issues related to social inequality and racism is a particularly enormous task."

Physical activity may be especially helpful in mitigating the stress associated with racial discrimination, and yet discrimination is a barrier to being physically active if you don't feel safe running in your neighborhood park!

Here are some ideas to support your right to safe and enjoyable outdoor physical activity.

- Prioritize safety. Your physical safety is most important. If you feel unsafe jogging in your current environment, consider finding a friend or family member to jog with you, joining a running group, and taking your phone with you for documentation. Seek out fitness groups, sports teams, or community centers that make clear on their website or brochures that they aim for inclusivity and belonging. And if you prefer outdoor exercise, are there parks or trails in your area that feel more inclusive and safe? Consider going at a time where there are more people around to be witnesses.

- Stay informed. Know your rights in situations involving racial profiling. Check out the *At Liberty Podcast* for ideas about how to respond if you believe you're being racially profiled. There are also numerous resources at ACLU.org. It's a great place to learn more about racial profiling, its impact, and strategies for addressing it.

- Advocacy and allyship: Build connections with others who share similar experiences within your community. Engage in discussions, activism, or advocacy efforts related to racial justice and equity in public spaces. On the ACLU website at aclu.org/action, there are a range of options, some that will take just a few minutes and others that will take some extra time.

It's not your personal responsibility to make your park a safe place to run; systemic change is needed. At the same time, physical activity is a great way to mitigate the negative stress associated with discrimination. I encourage you to keep finding creative ways to move, while at the same time practicing self-compassion. It's hard to move in a world that is unjust.

Rethinking Movement
Many Movement Communities

While having a running partner or group is a quick solution for being and feeling safer exercising in your area, there are also many organizations actively working on accessible movement communities for people of color. Some are online platforms full of practical tips, personal stories, and regular meetups for anyone wanting to get outside for a walk, run, hike, and more, without feeling like they don't belong in a space.

Over and over again, community can help us get moving. Community can mean finding an exercise buddy or a running group to join for a "safety in numbers" effect. It can also mean finding online communities that are working hard to normalize fitness and outdoor activities specifically for people of color (e.g., Afro Outdoors, Girl Trek, Melanin Basecamp), including making regular old outside exercises—going to the park, taking a jog through a neighborhood, hiking in a national park—safe and inclusive for all.

Another way to reach for community is through story. Read movement memoirs of other folks who've physically negotiated, and continue to negotiate, racist landscapes (literal and metaphorical) because movement was important to them, like *Running While Black* by Alison Désir, *The Unlikely Thru-Hiker* by Derick Lugo, *Spirit Run* by Noe Alvarez, *Pack Light* by Shilletha Curtis, and *The Home Place* by J. Drew Lanham.

While this barrier is entirely different from any other barriers, the physiological need to move your body continues to exist despite it. Movement belongs to you. Your physical and mental health depend on it. Racially inclusive fitness facilities and classes exist. Find them and use them. The rest of the work—systemic change—isn't yours to lift alone; it belongs to everyone.

Reason 38: I loathe my boring, flat, nearly treeless suburban neighborhood for any kind of walking. It's zoned such that to get anywhere you must walk along a narrow lane right next to a busy road. No sidewalks along said busy road, which is dangerous. I'd have to drive to get to a nice walking trail with trees.

It's de-motivating for sure when your neighborhood doesn't support walking. And we hope that it being boring and flat doesn't deter you from taking that walk! One way to work with this is to practice getting flexible with your attention.

Our attention is like a flashlight, and we can always choose where to point it. We tend to regularly point our attention flashlight towards the things we "loathe," further building up the story about how much, for example, we hate our neighborhood—and our loathing only grows brighter!

Attention Shifting

One way to decrease our loathing of something is to shine our attention-light on things we enjoy. So try taking a walk through your boring, flat, nearly treeless suburb, and see how many other things you notice about your space beside it being treeless. Literally count them!

Can you notice how it feels in your body to take a brisk walk? The pretty clouds in the sky? The music you're listening to? The color of the sunset or sunrise? The decorations in the storefront windows? The information being shared on your favorite podcast? How cozy you feel in your jacket? The flowers or birds in your neighborhood? The neighbor you haven't seen in a while?

If you're searching for even more to pay attention to, invite a friend to walk with you so you have a relationship and good conversation to pay attention to.

Behavioral Shifting

Behavioral flexibility is another way to gain more freedom and agency when you feel trapped.

Variety can make things more enjoyable and tolerable (remember psychological richness on pages 59–60). Maybe some days you drive to a lovely tree-lined walking path, and other days you walk some of those small treeless streets that don't go anywhere.

Ultimately, you have a choice: to not walk and feel badly about it, or to walk and allow it to be what it is—"This is where I live and there's a convenient walk right here." You just might find that by shifting your attention, switching things up a bit, and practicing acceptance, you'll loathe the walking experience of your neighborhood a little less. Or maybe you still hate it, and you walk anyway. We are fine with both, and your body will be too.

Rethinking Movement
Streets That Go Nowhere

So much of what we do for exercise is movement that goes nowhere. Treadmills or stationary bikes don't get you to and from work. You can swim a hundred laps and get out right where you started. Picking up weights is just lifting and lowering something for the sake of lifting and lowering it, and you can jump rope for twenty minutes and never go higher than a handful of inches. Does every walk we take need to go somewhere?

I (Katy) have walked what feels like a million miles, in different parts of the world, along beautiful beaches, in the wilderness, through engaging cityscapes full of street art and coffee shops and people watching. And in my top three favorite walking routes of all time is a three-mile route in a suburban neighborhood I used to live in. While the route went

193

nowhere—I couldn't walk for any practical reasons—I was always able to travel and explore the length of my mind, which is one of the reasons I like to walk so much. (Other bonuses: I didn't need to add any time to my day to get to and from my walk, and if something came up that cut into my walk time, I could simply adjust the out-and-back and still fit some amount of walking into my day.)

There are certainly benefits to being surrounded by beauty or interesting views when you're walking when it comes to motivation, but by focusing on other positives—a chance to get outside, have a dose of sunlight, listen to an audiobook, podcast, or music without interruption, get body movement, connect with what's going on with your immediate community— you're likely to find a new source of motivation that expands your toolkit.

7

It's Hard to Move with Other People

In earlier chapters we have noted some of the many benefits of moving with others. We are more motivated when we move in community. Dynamic relationships can boost our mood, support our brain health, and keep us accountable. And having movement buddies makes it easier to slot movement into daily life, because you're not having to choose between physical activity and relationships. But what if you just can't get the ones you love to move with you? Worse yet, what if your loved ones are preventing you from moving?

Maybe you're hopeful this chapter will show you how to motivate others to start exercising; in fact, our primary message will continue to be that, ultimately, you can only control yourself. Focus on your values. Use your cognitive flexibility skills so you're not swayed by guilty thoughts like *taking a walk is selfish* or thrown off by teens who won't leave their gaming beanbag to exercise. Practice acceptance—sometimes going against the sedentary grain is uncomfortable, and you have to move when your dog goes on strike, your new baby needs attention, and your spouse won't budge. You now have the psychological flexibility skills to move around and with these obstacles, so open up and keep your commitment to the bigger reasons you want to move.

And, okay, we also have some tricks and tips for getting others to move with you, but there's a catch. You might have to get *even more* flexible.

There's nothing better than everyone being on the same page movement wise, but here's a pop quiz for you: Do you truly want everyone to be on the same page, or do you want everyone to be on *your* page? If you're trying to force people onto your page, you aren't going to move very far.

The psychological tools we use to align with another person's perspective (instead of trying to get them to align with ours) include empathy, perspective-taking, and attunement—being fully present and responsive to another person's emotional state. This requires us to understand our inner world (why is it so frustrating when people won't move with us?), and also to join theirs (what is blocking them from moving?). To join "their world," we need to practice nonjudgmental acceptance. How can you approach your loved one with curiosity, and without trying to change them?

In this section, you'll practice staying open to different perspectives, and being willing to give up being "right" in order to connect—to others and to the movement you want and need. Maybe you need to get on their page...or maybe you need to create a brand new page that fits everyone just right.

Reason 39: My dog goes on strike if I try to walk her more than a trip around the block. She just stops and lies down. I end up dragging her on the leash around the park, which isn't fun for either of us.

Dear everyone, even if you don't have a dog, we suggest reading through our answer and replacing "dog" with the loved one of your choice. Yes, we're serious.

When I (Diana) was in graduate school for clinical psychology, the first textbook I was assigned to read was called *Don't Shoot the Dog! The New Art of Teaching and Training.* Written by animal trainer Karen Prior, the book describes the principles and practices of teaching new behaviors—without using threats, force, punishments, or guilt trips. Why are beginning psychologists given a book on animal training? Because all animal behavior follows the same simple behavioral principles—we need to be cued to do a behavior, we repeat behaviors that are reinforced, and punishment is not very effective. The committed action process in ACT leans on this science of behavior change.

In his book *Atomic Habits,* James Clear describes the Four Laws of Behavior Change: Make the habit you want to develop obvious, make it attractive, make it easy, and make it satisfying. You can use these steps to get your dog (and yourself) walking without having to do so much dragging. Don't forget, it takes a little perspective-taking—what's it like to be your dog?

1. Make it obvious. Environmental cues like keeping your leash in the same spot, walking at the same time every day, strapping on your fanny pack of treats, or saying a command ("Let's go for a walk!") will prepare your dog to walk. I (Diana) keep all our walking supplies in a drawer

in our kitchen, along with doggie bags and treats. As soon as that drawer opens, my dog comes running! She knows what we are up to because we have made it obvious it's time to walk.

2. Make it attractive. Make your walk appealing by reinforcing your dog as you head out. You can use reinforcements like dog treats and verbal praise (no pup can resist a high pitched "Good puppy!") or bring along their favorite tennis ball, frisbee, or dog toy. Adjust your walk to match their pace some of the time. Let them stop and sniff. Let them sprint and stop and sprint again. (That's good for both of you; more on this below.) Verbalize the fun you are having out loud—remember that your dog wants to please you, and the tone of your voice tells them you are having a good time with them.

3. Make it easy. In order to grow new behavior, you need to make it achievable and easy to get going. Make sure your dog is hydrated and not too hot before you leave. Make it easier for your dog to walk next to you than it is to lie down by shortening your leash. Follow a predictable path. Make it easier for yourself by committing to not battling your dog, even shortening your walk if necessary.

4. Make it satisfying. Make the new habit of walking with your dog rewarding for both of you. When you arrive home, give your dog a chance to lie down and rest. Get on the floor with them, cuddle, and enjoy the satisfaction of coming home from a nice walk outdoors. Celebrate your efforts together!

If after all that your dog still doesn't want to walk very far, you can get flexible and take two walks—one for the dog, one for the human. Your dog's lack of interest isn't a good reason to not get longer walks for yourself. Your dog can strike, and you can still go for a walk.

Rethinking Movement
Dogs Just Want to Have Fun

We can all learn a lot from dogs. I (Katy) started walking my dog a few times every day when she was quite young. Because I walked everywhere—to the grocery store, to the post office, through the neighborhood with my kids, and on longer hikes—she became an avid walker too. As a heeler she's bred to be a working dog on a farm or ranch, so she naturally prefers a lot of movement, and walking a lot isn't an issue for her. But dogs (and people for that matter) aren't *only* walkers. There are other types of movement that make up a dog's perfect movement plan. In addition to a lot of walking-type traveling movement, heelers are bred for speed and agility, and their bodies need to do things like sprint and stop on a dime before jetting off in a different direction. Agility-type exercise is part of a dog's healthy movement diet. It's also in a dog's DNA to bound and jump around and do their dog version of wrestling. And a dog's muscles, joints, and bones aren't the only parts of their body that need these kind of movements; their brains are also wired for the focus it takes to do them and the achievement of being successful at them. Playful movements like these are not only nutritious, they are satisfying to a dog.

After almost a year of heading out on the same mile-long walk to the post office, my movement-loving dog sat down at the end of the road one day and let me know she didn't want to go. Then she did it the next day, and the next, and the next. I tried forcing her a couple of times, but that didn't work out. I started leaving her behind, which wasn't great either, because she still needed more movement. One day, she saw me head out for the walk and ran and grabbed the soccer ball and dropped it at my feet. I finally understood. *I want to move my body, and I'd like to be with you, but this walk is boring. Can we move in this other way?*

After ten minutes of dog soccer play (me kicking and chasing the ball—movements that are very good for my hips and legs as well—while she tried to trap it or sprint after ones that got by her) she was ready to walk with me. Sometimes I'd carry the ball for the first part of the walk and play along the way. She was perfectly willing to come on a walk if there was going to be something she liked occurring along the way. Since then I've also started to play soccer (or frisbee or chase or wrestle) with her for a few times a day for a handful of minutes in the mornings and evenings, because this movement is not only good for her body, it's good for my body too. It makes her life more interesting and deepens our relationship.

This might not be your exact situation, but the point stands—just because your dog doesn't want to go for a walk doesn't mean they don't want to move with you. Dogs are people too, and they have their own preferences and needs. If they've been left alone most of the day with little interaction or movement, they might adapt to being under-stimulated and develop general malaise. Or they might find taking the same walk, the same direction, at the same pace (*your* pace, which, depending on the dog's size, might be forcing them to walk slower than their natural baseline gait, which is more like a trot) boring and uncomfortable.

Meet your dog partway. Offer an energetic play and snuggle/wrestling session that you use for your own warmup before heading out all alone on the walk that works for *your* body. Try reversing the route, going off trail, or changing the time of day you walk to see if there's a change in your dog's interest. Instead of walking at the park, once you get there let them chase a ball or stick or frisbee in between you doing squats or push-ups. In addition to walking time, physically engage with your dog more often, but for short, playful bouts that say "I see what you like and need, and even if I don't love this movement, it gets my body more of the movements it needs and it's good for you, and I love you, so I'm happy to do it."

Did we mention that this advice can be also used for kids, including teens? Dogs (and kids for that matter) can be excellent personal trainers. Their instincts for movement might be more intact than yours, and if you follow their lead, they can help you mix up your own movement diet and get out of a ruff. I mean rut.

Reason 40: I have five children and no one to help me get them outside, no one to help focus on child safety or hold the baby. There's so much to explore outside, but I don't feel like I have the capacity to facilitate it alone. The baby is too heavy for a wrap but too little to walk alongside. So we just don't move. It's suffocating.

That sounds like a lot to manage, and, yes, five kids inside can get a bit chaotic and suffocating! At the same time, don't underestimate yourself as a wise, skillful parent. You take care of five kids every day, which means you have a lot of experience in creating child safety, holding babies while multitasking, and facilitating kid-friendly experiences. Maybe you have done this in the airport, at a holiday gathering, or at a friend's birthday party.

An outdoor adventure is simply a new context in which to practice these skills you already have. In psychology, taking a skill we already have and applying it to a new setting is called *generalization*. Let's get some perspective here! You already know how to manage five kids in a lot of different scenarios, and this next step isn't the big leap you might think.

When you feel overwhelmed, breaking things down into smaller steps can really help. When you have a minute and (some of?) the kids are napping or settled with a game, make yourself a cup of tea and pull out your notebook.

What Are Your Strengths?

Start by looking at what you do well and what you know how to do, and then we can work towards generalizing it to the outdoors.

What are your greatest strengths as a parent? What is your zone of parental genius? Are you a powerhouse at organization? Skilled at being present when your kids show complex emotions? Perhaps your superpower is commitment—you are persistent in making plans happen. Maybe you are super patient, or great at storytelling or making up creative games.

If you need help zeroing in on these, just consider the many ways you are already keeping your kids safe, setting boundaries, and corralling them when they are headed in five directions. Think of other times when what you want to do with your kids seems impossible and you make it possible. What do you already do around your house that works? Do you have the older kids help the younger ones? Set up physical barriers around the new crawlers and walkers? Use games to help kids learn boundaries? Use praise or other forms of positive reinforcement? Write all your best parenting skills down.

Make sure you get specific. For example, I (Diana) have a superpower of emotional sensitivity. I can tell when a kid is about to hit their limit. A skill I have leaned on for years is to notice when they are getting flustered and ask them if they want to go to the garden with me to pick some herbs for dinner. We usually stay out longer than expected and get a chance to chat, and their mood shifts by the time we return.

What do you do that works with your kids? Consider how you may apply that same skill when you are moving outside.

The next step is to see how you might generalize these superpowers and skills to your outdoor adventures and make a plan.

Rethinking Movement
Your Outdoor Movement Plan

Being outside with a group of kids can feel overwhelming, but making a plan is one way to decrease some of the risk you're perceiving.

First, identify the outdoor spaces you feel safe to explore. There are many ways for you and your kids to engage with the great outdoors, and not all of them need to be moving far distances on foot. You just need a parcel of greenspace that works for your comfort and ability level. There might be an accessible solution right out your front (or back) door, like a yard, park, or sports field, where the space is open and you can keep an eye on all your kids at once. If you feel better with tighter boundaries, look for options with fences that do some of the herding for you. Or, do what nature school teachers do and use a portable set of bright orange cones to mark off smaller areas within larger ones, and show kids the areas they're expected to stay within.

Practice outdoor ways of communicating, so you can stay in contact despite kids moving farther away from you. Coaches, who often take large groups of kids outside on their own, don't spend a lot of time screaming after kids. Get a whistle and teach your kids to return to home base when they hear it. I (Katy) have a set of family "bird calls" (another trick taken from our time in nature school) that allow us to communicate quickly without having to shout or even see where everyone is. A crow call means "Stop what you're doing." A quail's "chi-ca-go, chi-ca-go" means "Come to me now." Make a game out of whistles or calls at first, to hone everyone's listening and responding skills. Practice in smaller spaces and test to see how far the kids can go and still return when they hear you calling. Move to larger areas when you feel ready.

Make sure you have the right gear. For kids too heavy to hold and easily fatigued from walking, a wagon makes a great ally in outdoor adventures. Not only can tired kids take a rest while you're on the move, other kids can take turns pushing and pulling and playing with the wagon. Even if you're going slow, or hardly going anywhere, you're all still getting lot of movement and outside time, which is the name of this game, and you're all building the skills you'll need to eventually go farther, faster.

Lean on others, too. This can be other adults who bring their own kids to an outdoor meetup (more kids, yes, but more adult eyes on everyone's kids, too) or older kids, ten to twelve years old, who can act as a parent helper for walks or outdoor games you've chosen. Look for outdoor group movement activities where you can stay and participate, but that you don't have to facilitate. Also, look for unconventional times for outdoor exploring. If there's more parental support in the evening, ditch your sit-down indoor kitchen table and pack the wagon (you got the wagon, right?) or a backpack with a simple picnic dinner you can snack on while adventuring together. Make this extra rich by inviting some other friends and families who have probably also been struggling to figure out how to make dynamic outdoor time happen.

When it comes to exploring outside, check in with what you're picturing, and consider letting that ideal go to make space for all the great times you haven't even imagined yet.

Reason 41: My teenagers won't move, they'll only game or be on their phones, and I sit there stewing about it.

Warning: This is a long answer. That's because teens are a special situation, with their mental, physical, and social development all happening at a breakneck pace, in a new modern context that parents can barely get their heads around. We both get a lot of questions about teens and screens and movement. You've been warned!

It can be tempting to tell your teen, "Get off your phone!" or threaten to throw the gaming console out the window (Diana's done both) when you see them lounging on their screens. However, battling your teen about their screen use is likely to backfire, and even worse, damage your relationship with them.

When you look more closely at your frustration, you will see that something you care about is driving it. You are stewing because you care. Anger is a form of energy, and what matters most is what you do with it. You can yell and threaten your kids, potentially damaging your relationship and influence; you can sit there stewing in your fury (not good for anyone, least of all you); or you can use that anger-energy to motivate you to move towards your values—like connecting with your kids, caring for your body, and helping them learn to care for theirs.

Get to Know Your Inner World

Get out your notebook and spend some time exploring your frustration. This exercise is modified from the work of Richard Schwartz, who wrote the book *No Bad Parts*, and it's a great way to take perspective on your inner experience. There are likely many parenting-teen parts inside you, not just a stewing part. You have a frustrated part and also a loving part, and a part that wants you and your teen to move. So let's explore these "parts."

Stewing part: What does your stewing part think about your kids on screens? Why does your stewing part care so much? What is important to your stewing part?

Loving part: What does your loving part think about your kids on screens? Why does your loving part care so much? What is important to your loving part?

Mover part: What does the part of you that wants you and your teen to move think? Why does your mover part care so much? What is important to your mover part?

Now, see if you can access a wise self that can hold all of these parts at the same time—we'll call it your wise parent self. What does your wise parent self say? Is there a way to act that aligns with your values, and also honors these parts?

Get to Know Your Teen's World

In the book *Behind Their Screens*, Dr. Emily Weinstein and Dr. Carrie James share the results of their study examining technology use and attitudes of over 3,500 teens. Their conclusion? The narrative that screens plus teens equals misery is overly simplistic. Adults are not seeing the full picture when it comes to understanding teens' screen use. For many teenagers, gaming and phones are their direct link to social connection, tools to navigate our world, and means to take important developmental risks. As adults, we can do a better job of learning how to work with our teens to stay physically active in our technology-dominant world. At the heart of your success in this is your connection with your teenager. Build a connection, listen more than you talk, be their coach, and help them learn from their own experience. Stop battling your teenager and learn more about why they play video games. Explore these different reasons they are on their screens with them to understand their perspective better. We've included some questions to get the conversation going. Remember, it's about perspective-taking, and attunement. What does your teen think and feel? It's time to ask!

Risk-taking needs. Are your teens playing Fortnite because they are seeking a little dopamine rush? During adolescence, the developing brain exhibits heightened reactivity within the reward center known as the ventral striatum. This neurological transformation fuels their curiosity for new experiences and an eagerness to explore the world around them. This brain adaptation plays a crucial role in motivating teenagers to seek independence. However, the impulse control center of a teenager's brain, located in the frontal lobe, is not yet fully matured. This dual dynamic makes adolescents more vulnerable to engaging in risky behaviors. Video games and the world of social media/messaging provide an environment where teenagers can experiment with and express this drive for risk-taking behavior and emotional expression.

Try capitalizing on this inclination by setting up ways for your teen to take measured physical risks that meet the needs of their brain and body at the same time. One thing that will get my (Diana's) two sons off screens and outside is building mountain bike jumps, then jumping them. This form of healthy risk-taking is exactly what teens need and often why they turn to video games—they want to feel the focus and adrenaline that come with being on the edge of danger.

Ask your teen a few questions about taking risks:

- What type of physical risks do you like to take? Paintball? Ice blocking down a big hill? Jumping off the pier?
- What makes you feel alive in your body?
- What makes you feel genuinely challenged?
- What new physical skills do you want to get better at?

Then actively support your teen's risk-taking:

- Build more risk-taking spaces in your home. For example, in our (Diana's) house we have rings hanging from the ceiling of our playroom and a basketball hoop over the TV. It's always a risk when the kid misses a shot!

- Encourage physical risk-taking in your outdoor space. Make risk-taking easily accessible. Roller blading in the driveway? Skateboarding off the kitchen steps? Hold your breath, and let them do it (with a helmet of course!).
- Incorporate technology into risk-taking. Teens love to video and track their risk-taking behavior. Strap a GoPro to their helmet or add Strava to their phone/watch to track their speed and distance. If they are interested in using technology to support movement, support them in it!

Get attuned to your teen's need to take risks, and give them lots of opportunities to feel like they are riding the edge of life and death (without really risking it), and give them some space to do it without your breathing down their neck. Let them feel adventurous and free and go take yourself on a walk (or whatever movement *your* body and brain need) and savor the fact that everyone is on the same page—being physically nourished in the best way for them.

Social needs. Some teens play video games to meet their social needs. When I (Diana) asked my fourteen-year-old son about what he likes about gaming, he said, "Because games are social, there is an aspect of a challenge, and you can play with your friends."

Adolescence is a developmental stage in which the significance of peers and social bonds becomes particularly pronounced. Video games, social media, and texting can be central ways teens maintain their social networks and engage with their friends, and it's likely your teen can tell when their screen use is social versus isolating. They know the difference between playing Zelda alone on a Friday night when everyone else is at a school dance and yelling and laughing while playing games with their best friends on a Saturday morning.

Ask your teen a few questions about their social needs:

- Which friends do you like talking with the most on your [Xbox/computer/phone/PlayStation]?

- What's fun about gaming/Snapchatting/making videos with your friends?
- Who's the best at [X game]? Whose social feed do you like to follow the most? Can you show me your favorite posts?
- Do you want to meet up with the friends you are playing with online in person?
- Need me to chauffeur you anywhere? I'm game!

Once you get an understanding of your kid's social needs, you can support them in building more in-person connections centered around movement.

Note: You cannot just skip to this part. You have to have connection with them first, and you have to understand what it is they love about their tech experiences. They can sniff your insincerity out a mile away, and will know if you're briefly feigning interest just to skip to the part where you tell them to move more.

Independence needs. As much as you might like to, you can't follow your kids to college. Soon enough they will be on their own to manage their screen use, and they are likely already craving some independence right now. Capitalize on this, and help them become their own technology police. Help them learn how to modulate their screen time so you don't have to. Ask your teens what they don't like so much about being on a screen. Then they'll be able to articulate for themselves feelings of getting sucked in and not doing other things they'd rather do, or the loneliness of playing alone and the difficulty of stopping even when it doesn't feel good.

Ask your teen:

- What are the things you like and what are the things you don't like so much about gaming/being on your phone/social media?
- How do you think we could up the stuff you like and decrease the stuff you don't like?
- How do you know when it's time to stop and take a break?
- What boundaries do you want to put on your screen time?

- How does it feel in your body when you are on screens?
  What about when you get off?

Encourage them to check in with their body regularly. Your teen can tell that they feel better when they move; their mood tanks when they sit all day at school, and getting active helps their focus, releases pent-up energy, and moves emotions through them.

Teens learn through experience; ask more questions than you give answers, and help them connect the dots without shaming, stepping in too soon, or acting like a know-it-all. And most importantly, be a model. Even when they are not moving, you still can. Your kids are watching what you do more than listening to what you say. If you are on your computer or phone telling them to get outside, they will see right through it. Instead put down your phone, and say out loud, "I can tell my body needs to move. I'm going to go outside and take a lap around the block." Be the change you want to see in your kids.

Rethinking Movement
Don't Forget the Fun

If you're trying to get kids to choose movement over an alternate reality where they don't have to obey everyday rules *or* the laws of gravity, movement needs to be enticing. Telling kids to "go play outside" can feel pretty pale (and dated) in the face of all brighter colors and sounds just a handful of inches from their face.

The good news is, bursts of movement are pleasing to teen brains, as are bursts of personal achievement. The easier these are to engage with, the more likely your teen will choose them repeatedly throughout the day. When my (Katy's) kids were small, it was challenging to meet both their all-day need for movement and our adult needs to get work and chores done. We simply couldn't get out to parks and play areas as much as the kids would have liked! Our solution was to bring exercise-y things into our home that we could strew about that promoted toddler-friendly balance, strength, and climbing challenges. Now that our kids are older, we continue to pepper fun and challenging movement opportunities throughout the home, making the choice to move easy to integrate. Place a mini-trampoline in the living room. Start jumping on it yourself, and ask your teens how long they think you can go without stopping. Then watch them push you off so they can see how long *they* can go without stopping. Wobble boards, rings and doorway pull-up bars, exercise balls, Pogo balls, and climbing holds up a wall are great ways to promote bursts of fun activity—no "exercise" or even going outside required.

Kids and teens will often come home looking for something challenging to do and find not much besides a computer to play on. Get a portable ping-pong set you can use on your dining room table and announce after dinner that it's time for a family playoff. Set up a few trick shots that have to be mastered before your teen can turn on the tech for more easily acquired dopamine hits.

All of us parenting children right now are doing so in unknown territory. We are the first generation of parents that have to negotiate the landscape of ubiquitous tech and screen time. Our fully formed brains struggle with our own tech boundaries, and we're even more worried about our kids, who are still in the process of developing their brains. And all the sitting and being inside is stressful for everyone involved. Share your value words with your teens and ask them to come up with their own set of values as well. Then collaborate and come up with a set of family values too, and use these as a way of framing good use practices around technology and movement in the home. And remember to have fun! Play is a wonderful portal into physical activity, and your teens can make great personal trainers when it comes to getting you out of your own activity comfort zone.

Finally, create family rituals around movement. Which rituals did you enjoy as a family growing up that you can bring to life now? Did you rake leaves together? Go on family walks? Dig in the garden? Walk after dinner? Walk to church on Sundays? Go camping for summer holidays? Skiing or skating for winter holidays? Commit to creating memories around moving together, even if your teen rolls their eyes at you as you go.

Reason 42: My partner hates to move. I can't get them on board to move with me.

We are sure that wanting to get your partner moving with you comes from a loving place. However, we also all know what it feels like when someone tries to get us "on board" with their agenda. We naturally push back! In order to get your partner moving, they will need reasons that are personal and relevant to them. One way to get at this is through motivational interviewing.

Motivational interviewing is a technique often used in therapy, healthcare, coaching, and education, where the goal is to support someone in exploring their own motivations and building commitment to positive change. Research has shown that motivational interviewing can be more effective than traditional advice-giving approaches, particularly when it comes to behaviors that are complex or difficult to change. While this tool is used in high-stakes scenarios like substance-use treatment facilities and even hostage negotiations, you can use it in your home too. Rather than pushing for change, or straight up nagging your loved one, you can simply ask questions that help them explore and articulate their personal thoughts and reasons to change.

Our guess is there is more nuance than just your partner "hates to move." They may have parts of them that want to move, and other parts that really resist it. Motivational interviewing allows for this type of ambivalence while also encouraging the parts of them that want to make positive changes.

Here are some ideas of how to apply motivational interviewing skills to encourage your partner to move their body more.

Stop pleading, complaining, and nagging. Probably the best way to get someone *not* to exercise is to shame, blame, or criticize them about it.

Reinforcement, not punishment, supports changes in behavior. So, your first step is to stop making things worse by nagging your partner to get on board. Instead, interview them, and use active listening to learn more about their experience. You might say:

- I want to know more about what not wanting to exercise is like for you.
- Do you want to move in other ways?
- What is hard about exercise or moving more for you?
- What do you hope for yourself?

When they respond, reflect back what you hear to make sure you are getting it right. Resist the urge to set them straight!

Develop discrepancy. It's likely that your partner isn't fully satisfied with how much they are moving either. Motivational interviewing capitalizes on this discrepancy between a person's actual behavior and how they want to behave by asking open-ended questions. You can highlight this discrepancy by asking questions like these:

- On a scale from 0 to 10, how satisfied are you with how much you are moving? What would make you feel more satisfied?
- It seems like there's a difference between where you are now and where you want to be. Tell me more about what would make you feel better about how you are moving.
- If a year from now you were closer to where you want to be in terms of moving your body, what would that look like?
- What would help you bridge the gap between where you are and where you want to be?

Roll with resistance. If your partner expresses resistance or defensiveness, avoid arguing or pushing them further away. Instead, gently acknowledge their feelings and validate their perspective. Try to understand the reasons behind their resistance without judgment. Let them be ambivalent, and roll with it. Remember, this is about attunement and active listening! You can try a few different approaches:

- Tell me more about why you hate to move.

- What are the good things and the not-so-good things about moving your body?

- Tell me about the part of you that doesn't want to move, and the part of you that does.

Elicit change talk. With all this questioning, you may start to notice the tide shift and your partner arguing for why they want to move more, how they need to move more. This is called *change talk* in motivational interviewing. When it happens, reinforce it! Highlight their reasons for wanting change and repeat them back. Affirm their strengths and remind them of the other times they have been successful at changing. For example:

- What I'm hearing you say is that you actually do want to move more, even if it doesn't always seem like it. Tell me more about a time when you liked moving.

- I guess I was wrong. Is it that you don't really hate moving, you just hate feeling forced to move? Or is it something else?

- I believe in you. I've seen you make changes and stick with them before, for example, when you...

- I remember when you took up pickleball last spring, how it was hard to get there in the beginning but then you loved the feeling of being with friends and the stress relief it brought.

Instead of trying to get your partner on board, step back and look at the board *with* them. You just may find, together, there are more creative, flexible ways to support your partner in exploring their own motivations for being more active (not yours!). With this type of questioning, you will support them in making the changes they want to make at their own pace.

Remember, it's about the changes *they* want to make, not the ones *you* want them to make. If you give your best interviewing skills a shot and it's still abundantly clear that your partner doesn't want to change, don't use up all your energy to force it.

Ultimately, your power is in getting yourself moving, and loving your partner as they are, not the partner you hope to turn them into. Seek to understand, but don't get stuck there—get up and move whether your partner comes along with you or not. That is the one thing you have under your control.

Rethinking Movement
Love and Hate

There are many people who hate exercise but love to move, or at least love some way of moving their body. Movement and exercise have become so muddled in our minds that whenever anyone mentions "getting active" or "staying in shape," we default to thinking of workouts, gym equipment, or types of movement done to get our heart rates up and our muscles burning. Many people don't enjoy fitness-type ways of moving, and might have forgotten there are ways of being physical they do enjoy: banging drums for two hours, playing a game of basketball, riding horses, throwing pottery, dancing to live music, working in the yard, building something outside, foraging for mushrooms, wrestling with the dog, carrying a squirmy toddler.

Ask your loved one some questions to expand and further deepen their exploration of movement, including ways of moving that sit outside of the fitness and health paradigm:

- What's your favorite movement memory (i.e., your most joyful, satisfying movement experience)? How was your body moving while you were making that memory?

- Which physical experiences do you miss, that you would like to do again?

- Are there things you want to do with your body (a three-day backpacking trip, tying your shoes without pain, going across the monkey bars) that you can't do now?

As you're interviewing, listen closely to the answer to see if you can identify ways your loved one likes to move—or even is moving—that you might not have considered.

I (Katy) found that, as my kids got older, they no longer wanted to move with me like they did when they were little. Diana gave me great insight, though, and pointed out that the movement I was inviting them to do (walk and hike—my favorite!) might not be the type of movement they found most interesting. Were there any movements they liked that I could try? It turns out my kids were inviting me to move all the time. Would I arm wrestle, could I hold their legs while they worked on backbends, how about a race across the parking lot, would I come play goalie while they fired soccer balls at my head? Because these movements weren't what I was imagining when trying to fulfill my daily need for *exercise*, I thought my kids didn't want to move. Once I started listening, I found they were asking me for movement just as often as I was asking them; our modes of movement just looked different. And I feel good about doing the movements they like with them, and the movements I like with myself.

By going through this process, maybe you'll find that there are ways of moving that allow you and your loved one to connect more deeply, and also get you moving outside of your comfort zone and help deepen your personal relationship with movement.

Reason 43: My partner and I just adopted a baby and I feel guilty taking time to exercise when I could be with them. At the same time I'm noticing that without my daily trip to the gym I'm getting more irritable and resentful.

Congratulations on your new baby! What a big change for you and your partner—bringing a baby home rearranges your whole life. Every baby is different and changes rapidly, so we often have to improvise as we go. And the psychological changes that come with having a baby can bring a heightened sense of interdependence. As a result, many parents feel torn between spending time with their family members (who probably need you!) and prioritizing their own wellbeing (you need you too!). We both still feel this way, and our babies are now so old they are growing facial hair!

These feelings might not ever really go away, because they are related to your values. Parental guilt points to your longing to be there for your kids and partner—to be a good caretaker because you love them. And resentment about having your "me" time taken up by piles of laundry and diaper changes points to you caring about yourself. On top of that, when you're sleep deprived, all of your feelings are heightened, and your brain's negativity bias is in full force. However, if you can dig under these feelings to find your values, you will discover a wonderful thing about being a parent—you care deeply, and you can act on what you care about anywhere (at the gym, in the grocery store parking lot while mixing formula, or during tummy time). To start, let's dig under your feelings a bit to explore the values that are driving them.

Explore Your Values

When your baby is taking a nap, get out your notebook and explore some of the values underneath these feelings. Write at the top the feelings you are having, for example, *Guilt* and *Resentment*. Then underneath write about the values driving those feelings. For example, you may be feeling guilty because you value responsibility (you feel a strong duty to prioritize your baby and partner's needs) or presence (you want to be emotionally and physically available for bonding with your baby). And you may be feeling resentful because you value social connection (time at the gym was also a chance to see friends and feel a sense of community) or promoting mental health (you care about balancing your mood with movement). Remember that there are many ways to live out your values—and if you can identify the values driving how you are feeling, then you can better meet them in flexible ways. There are a lot of ways to express your values of responsibility, presence, social connection, and promoting mental health that don't involve going to the gym during this tender time in your family.

Diana's journey

I (Diana) first learned about Katy's work when I had a toddler and a new baby and was struggling with postpartum depression. The gym and yoga classes were an essential part of my mental health program before kids, but with a colicky baby and a strong maternal need to not leave him, I had to find more flexible ways to move. My partner and I would put Katy's podcast on in the morning while making breakfast (her cheery voice always improved my mood) and took some of her movement classes online in the evenings. I still remember lying on the ground with my legs in a "V" on the wall and a baby crawling on me. We also started listening to Shawn Stevenson's *The Model Health Show* and got some ideas for exercising from home. We bought a medicine ball that we threw back and forth, set up a battle rope outside next to our sandbox, and did planks in our living room while our baby had tummy time. As we babyproofed our house, we made it more movement rich too—we made a lot of room for our baby to safely crawl about, and for us to do bear crawls alongside him. We were so gung-ho we even cut the legs off our dining room table so we could sit on the floor together. I didn't have to give up my value of moving for mental health or my value of being there for my cognitively flexible, and the Nutritious Movement perspective helped with that.

Things have changed a lot since then (I now go to an exercise class to throw medicine balls and I'm back to doing yoga at my favorite studio), but I look back on those years with pride. It was hard, but we were psychologically flexible enough to keep moving, and I literally crawled my way out of postpartum depression.

Live Out Your Values

Once you identify your values, you can use other psychological flexibility processes to support you in living them out. Below are a few ideas.

Make it about "us." Shift your perspective from *me* to *we*. Your wellbeing is intertwined with your baby's and your partner's. You are a family system. When talking about movement with your family, use words like *we* and *us*, instead of *me* and *you*. Have an open conversation with your partner about how you are feeling. For example, "Let's work together to find a way that we can get more of our movement needs met in the day. We will be better parents because of it." This helps everyone recognize that your wellbeing is not separate.

Accept change with self-compassion. Your routine is likely going to need to adapt to accommodate your new role as a parent. When we hold on too tightly, trying to keep things the same, we are the opposite of psychologically flexible. Be patient with yourself as you navigate this transition period, and expect it to keep changing! Practice willingness, and be open to the uncomfortable feelings that come with change. Just because it's uncomfortable doesn't mean it's bad! Make space for your feelings, and practice self-compassion. You can say things like "It's understandable I feel this way. This is hard." Use the same tone of voice for yourself that you use to soothe your baby.

Think creatively. Step back from some of your mind's rules about what counts as movement and consider all the new ways you are moving with your baby that you never moved before. Bending, twisting, carrying, and crawling are all beneficial movements. Are there favorite gym moves you can bring home? See this as an opportunity to try new things like online classes, park exercise classes, home workouts, or shorter workouts interspersed throughout your day. Look for opportunities to involve your baby in your exercise routine, such as going for walks together in a stroller, dancing in music class, wearing your baby as you do housework, or doing baby-friendly workouts at home.

Engage alloparents. The ultimate form of self-compassion is remembering that you're not alone. Turn to others to help support you in parenting. Alloparenting is when caregiving is shared with non-parent providers. It's part of our evolutionary history, and research suggests cooperative parenting facilitates language, intelligence, and social emotional learning. By the age of three, over 90 percent of American children have experienced regular alloparental care. And research suggests that alloparenting leads to human females expending 14–19 percent less childcare effort across their lifetime compared to species that don't engage in alloparenting (which is most mammals).

It benefits you and your child when you share the load with others. Make a list of people who could be alloparents for your baby, and consider an exchange. Remember that alloparenting provides opportunities for your child to meet new people, strengthen bonds, and engage in a variety of stimulating activities they can't get with just you!

By finding ways to adapt to your new role as a parent, accepting the changes that come with it, and being flexible in your approach to movement, you can care for both yourself and your family. Remember that your wellbeing benefits your family, and your family's wellbeing benefits you; they are not separate, and it's possible to support both.

Rethinking Movement
Dynamic Rest, Active Alone Time

Becoming a mother and the corresponding loss of my (Katy's) personal exercise time was a pivotal movement in my career as a biomechanist and ultimately shaped the way I understand movement and teach about it today. I kept pondering this question: How could getting adequate movement, which is a biological necessity, be at such odds with everyday parts of life, like tending children—also a biological necessity? It didn't make sense to me from an evolutionary perspective, and I have been working on this question for well over a decade now, trying to find the movements in daily life that are much more compatible with all the other things that need to get done.

Every age and stage in life can impact our physical activity levels, and becoming a new parent is no exception. Research shows that up to half of regularly exercising adults drop their level of physical activity once they start raising kids, and this decrease is still apparent five years later. And P.S., mothers come in dead last when it comes to physical activity efficacy (our belief about our ability to successfully engage in exercise), even after diseased and frail elderly populations. It's no wonder. Taking care of young children is a full-time job alongside all the other full-time jobs we do. Exhausting! We're another human's arms and legs and eyes and ears so much of the time. Caretaking is physical. Our one body is doing a lot of the work for two (or three—talking to you, parents of twins!).

But here's a shift in perspective: The physical aspects of tending babies and toddlers are why, further research shows, new parents actually become *less* sedentary than they were before. While they do experience a steep decrease in their moderate and vigorous activity (often the stuff done at the gym or other places we went when we had free time), they sit less and have increased levels of light activity. Kids can keep you active in an entirely different way from before!

When I found myself in this situation, I kept thinking of our ancestors and how they met their needs for moderate to vigorous physical activity, and I realized that I could spend more time carrying my kids while walking for more intensity. When picking them up and setting them down dozens of times every day, I recognized "this is lifting weights" and started to pay attention to my form to really feel my muscles working well. I picked physical ways of playing with my kids (and I still do this now) and worked in stretching, strength, and sprints! Instead of feeling exhausted from just parenting, I reframed my fatigue and recognized that a least some of it was coming from getting more continuous movement throughout the day; knowing this made me feel less trapped by my new role (see the hotel worker study on pages 72–73 for more on why this perspective change is helpful in many ways!).

Lean into these new movement opportunities, even trying to expand them, and savor this time. When the littles stage is done, you'll feel a lot of the activity naturally built into your caretaking day slip away, and you'll even miss it. Never was my arm strength so easy to maintain without exercise!

None of this is meant to dissuade you from working on a plan to get you back to the gym. But your need to get there might be less about getting that daily dose of vigorous exercise, and more about taking a break. Parents need breaks, and our society's lack of community/alloparenting structure can make getting them quite difficult.

For me (Katy) the gym has always been a space for both movement and respite. Exercise was how I stepped away from work and relationships to just focus on myself for an hour. By not going to the gym when I had very young babies, I was missing out on *two* of my needs. That all being said, physical activity doesn't require a gym, and neither does a break. There can be ways of getting both things you need in a new way. Ask yourself (and write down your answer in your notebook!): If you were able to meet all your physical needs, even the vigorous ones, while being with your loved ones, what would you choose to do for a break? For me, even after moving with my kids, I will almost always choose doing some additional, focused movement work alone when I can, because that's what makes me feel my best. Your version of a break could look like reading in a hammock, taking a cooking class, getting a massage, or going to a book club or other social meetup.

Staying physically active throughout life is like working on a Rubik's Cube. Getting the colors on one side can mess up the symmetry on the other side, but we know there's a solution we're working towards, where more and more areas become organized. You're juggling a lot right now. You likely need rest, a break, and movement. These can all fit into our life most days, but they're just going to look different for you right now because your life is different. By focusing on making your family connection time as movement-rich as possible, you'll ultimately have more opportunities to choose the activities that make you feel like yourself when they arise.

Reason 44: Every time I try to get down on the floor to do my very specific and very helpful physical therapy exercises, either one of my children or the cat gets right on top of me, making it a lot more difficult.

Children and cats! Sounds like a fun floor to be on, and it can also pose a challenge when you are trying to be very focused on your therapeutic movements.

There's a place for acceptance here—not every physical therapy session will be as perfect as you want. This is also a place for committed action and setting some limits. When you need to focus on specific exercises, communicate that to your kids and find some time alone, maybe taking yourself into a different room. Doors can be closed to keep out the cats while you meet your movement needs. For less specific exercises, you might share the space and let your kids practice alongside you. You'll be modeling how to care for our bodies with movement, and spending time connecting (a stack!). You might find that after just a few minutes of attention, the kids will feel attended to and move on. Cats, on the other hand, may need to be moved to another room. If that's the case you will need to practice some acceptance of their protesting meows, while you finish up what you need to do. The key here is acceptance. There's no way around things being difficult, but hey, when you shift your perspective a little, you might also see positive elements—your cats and kids love you and want to be around you! That's a wonderful thing to savor.

Rethinking Movement
Get Down On It, Get Down On It

The floor might be the best piece of exercise equipment in our home. Not only can you do lots of cool movements once you're down there, just getting down and up again is an exercise in itself! Despite all those benefits, the amount of time adults tend to spend down there is pretty small. When you do get down to kid-and-pet level, that's exciting news for them, and excitement is physical! *Let's play! Let's wrestle! Scratch my ears! Rub my belly!* Which is different from how you're seeing the event: time to get down on the ground for the very *focused*, very *serious*, very *responsible* physical therapy session. Same floor, different page.

Take some of the excitement out of the room by making the floor exercise event less novel. Get down on the floor a few times a day, especially when you have nothing else to do down there but get some unstructured movement in with your kids and pets. Double the amount of time you get down on the floor "to do your exercises," but save one of those times for a less serious format. Ask your kids to correct your form, or film your routine. Let them know what you're doing and why. Now you're not only moving together and connecting, there's education happening too. When they have an issue, they'll be more inclined to consider movement as medicine. (My soccer-playing kids now ask me for a stretch for their sore bits after a game, and that's a result of the family culture we've created around movement as a tool for healing!) Create a game of stretch, strength, and balance challenges. Have your kids do one of your moves and then have them give you one of theirs to try.

By changing your relationship with the floor, you won't end up with exactly double the physical therapy time, but you'll log more physical therapy exercise time than before, and you'll get more total movement as well. It also means movement for your wrestling buddies and more connection with them too.

I Want to Move My Body And...

We picked forty-four reasons that choosing physical activity is difficult, but we know there are hundreds more we could have addressed. Our hope is that as you've read this book, you've begun to see the underlying solutions that emerge from our examples and can tailor them to your specific situation, even if it's not here. What's more, as you read through them, you likely generated some of your own creative solutions. We hope that you continue to customize these solutions to your own life, and continue this conversation with others as you walk, swim, stretch, skip, and bike about your day.

Our overarching goal with this book is to open everyone's minds, hearts, and bodies when it comes to movement. We are all different, *and* we are all humans with bodies that yearn to move. Remember, it's normal for minds and contexts to get in the way of moving your body, and you can use your heart, hands, and feet anyway. We hope that you take what you learned here and use it to build a more movement-rich and psychologically flexible life.

Below is a summary sheet for the psychological flexibility processes you learned about, along with a short description that sums up how to apply them to your personal movement blocks.

PROCESS	TAKEAWAY
KNOW YOUR VALUES	Remember what is most important to you and how you want to show up. Focus more on the process of living out your movement values than you do the outcome.
FLEXIBLE THINKING	Step back from self-sabotaging, critical, and unhelpful thoughts when it comes to movement. Notice thoughts, but don't act on them.
ACCEPT DISCOMFORT	Open up to and make space for discomfort when it comes to movement. Let go, loosen your grip, and allow.
TAKE PERSPECTIVE	Take perspective on yourself, and your self-stories. Take a broader view on movement, and see your movement as connected to something bigger than just you.
BE PRESENT	Be here now, in your body, in this moment.
TAKE COMMITTED ACTION	Make a move, make it attainable, and make it a habit.
PRACTICE SELF-COMPASSION	Encourage yourself to move with kindness and a commitment to your wellbeing. See your wellbeing as inherently connected to the wellbeing of others.

While the Rethinking Movement sections hold a wide range of practical solutions, there are also tenets of movement that show up again and again, that you can keep in mind.

Any movement is better than no movement at all. If you find yourself getting tripped up because the "shape" of your movement session isn't what you expected, consider flexing to a different way of moving your body right now. Staying psychologically flexible doesn't mean you'll *never* be able to get the exact movement session you want, but that you won't let perfectionism get in the way. Movement is like food, remember? We all have foods we love, but we don't expect to have our favorite meal multiple times a day or even multiple times a week. The key is to develop your palate—learn to tolerate and even enjoy many different foods—so you're nourished throughout the day, every day. The same goes for movement.

Take an action, any action at all, to get started. It takes more energy to get started moving than it does to keep on moving. In physics, *inertia* is an object's tendency to resist changes in its motion. As physical beings, we're always dealing with inertia—this "thing" that's trying to keep us doing what we're already doing. While inertia might seem to be the enemy of movement, ultimately it's an ally. Once you start moving, now you're moving—and inertia will work to *keep* you moving. If you've gleaned some ideas from this book about simple movements you can start with, pick the easiest to start doing right away. Maybe it's getting out of the chair and onto the floor to sit and read this book in a different shape. Maybe it's quickly tapping out a social media post that says, "Looking for an early morning walking buddy, want to start this week." Maybe it's throwing this book down and walking out the front door to take a seven-minute walk right now. You're not even going to change your clothes. (Do it! We'll wait.) You know the saying "mind over matter"? This is speaking to inertia! Your matter will tend to just keep on doing as it does; we need the mind to step in first, and let the matter follow. That said, we can't always *think* our way to moving more. We often need our thoughts to move out of the way first. In the case of "I know I should exercise, but," we're better to update the saying: "a compassionate, flexible, and present mind over matter."

Movement belongs to you. Movement is for every body. The need for it is written in our DNA. And, just like the nutrients in a food diet, we can customize our "movement nutrients" depending on what we need the most. We can have movement snacks and movement meals that work for our bodies and lives. But wait, there's more! If we take a lesson from Italian food culture, food—and movement, for this example—doesn't have to only be about *nutrients*. We can take great joy and pleasure from how we move our bodies, too. We can move a certain way or pick a mode of exercise *just because it feels good*. Even if exercise isn't your jam, you can still have a movement-rich life.

Community and movement go together. Movement belongs to you, but your movement is also part of the world. We currently live in a novel time, where movement has been removed from much of society's inner workings…and this shift towards sedentary culture has not been without consequences. Many of the issues we face—personal, social, and environmental—are affected by how little movement is now required to get things done. Oftentimes clearing a movement hurdle takes other people sharing the work of daily living. It takes sharing childcare: "I'll watch your kids while you go take a run. And bonus, while watching your kids, I'll take them to a park and we'll get some movement too." It takes reaching out to others: "I'd like to move my body more. Here's when I'm available/what I need. Does anyone want to do this with me?" It takes reclaiming some of the labor movement we've outsourced. Exercise doesn't grow on trees, but physical activity can. Do you have a helping hand (and helping arms, legs, and core muscles) to offer the individuals and larger communities around you that need physical volunteering? Can you put some of your movement towards a garden that helps feed your family or community? Plant some flowers to feed the pollinators? In short (a funny thing to write at the end of a long book), **your movement matters**. Your movement matters to your body, to your family, and to your community. If this tenet feels overwhelming when you read it, simply go back and reread the movement tenets above: everything counts, do what you love, in whatever amount you can manage right now.

You can lack motivation, be uncomfortable, not have enough time, feel the constant pull of a device, feel embarrassed, have no one to join you, and *all of the things*.

And you can move anyway.

References

To save paper and because you'll be accessing these sources online anyway, we've put chapter-by-chapter references and links for *I Know I Should Exercise, But...* online at uphill-books.com/IKISresources.

Index

About the Authors

Diana Hill, PhD, is a clinical psychologist and an internationally recognized expert in Acceptance and Commitment Therapy (ACT) and compassion. As the host of the *Wise Effort* podcast and author of *The Self-Compassion Daily Journal*, *ACT Daily Journal*, and the upcoming *Wise Effort*, Diana helps individuals and organizations cultivate psychological flexibility to lead fulfilling and impactful lives.

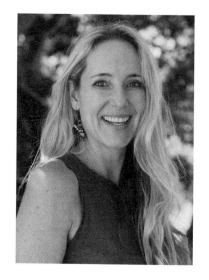

With over twenty years of meditation and yoga experience, Diana combines her deep personal practice with the latest psychological research to make wellbeing approachable and relevant to everyday life. Her work has been featured by NPR, *The Wall Street Journal*, *Woman's Day*, *Real Simple*, and other media outlets and she contributes regularly to Insight Timer, Mindful.org, and *Psychology Today*.

When not walking and talking with therapy clients, you'll find Diana digging in her garden, beekeeping, and taking sunrise ocean swims with her two boys.

Katy Bowman, M.S., is a biomechanist, movement teacher, and bestselling author of books that have changed the way many move and think about their need for movement. Her eleven books, including the groundbreaking *Move Your DNA*, have sold more than 300,000 copies in English and been translated into 16 languages worldwide.

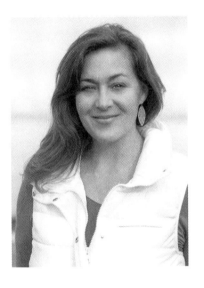

Named one of Maria Shriver's "Architects of Change" and an America Walks "Woman of the Walking Movement," Bowman teaches movement globally and speaks about sedentarism and movement ecology to academic and scientific audiences. Her work is regularly featured by national and international media including *The New York Times, The Guardian,* NPR, CBC Radio, *Seattle Times, Good Housekeeping, Outside, The Joe Rogan Experience,* and *The TODAY Show.* She has also worked with companies like Patagonia, Nike, and Google as well as a wide range of non-profits and other communities to create greater access to her "movement as nutrition" message.

Founder of the movement education company Nutritious Movement and host of the *Move Your DNA* podcast, Bowman lives in Washington State, where she spends as much time as she can moving outside with her family.

What Should I Read Next?

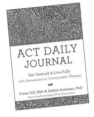

The **Act Daily Journal** *covers the six core processes of Acceptance and Commitment Therapy (ACT)—including mindfulness, acceptance, and values-based living. It also covers self-compassion, to help you roll with life's punches.*

The Self-Compassion Daily Journal *offers powerful writing prompts grounded in acceptance and commitment therapy (ACT), mindfulness, and compassion-focused therapy (CFT) to help you cultivate kindness and forgiveness toward yourself.*

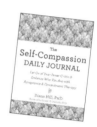

Watch for **Wise Effort** *(forthcoming 2025), a science-backed approach to shifting your most precious resource—your energy—to stop feeling depleted and reconnect with your inherent genius.*

If your movement hurdles include children and family, **Grow Wild** *is the book for you. Get everyone moving together, joyfully. Includes full-color photos to inspire movers of all ages.*

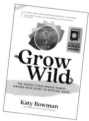

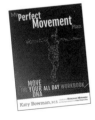

Once you're over your mental hurdles you'll need a plan. **My Perfect Movement Plan** *helps you figure out your "movement why," identify your missing moves, and make a movement plan you can stick to, right now.*

Ready for "movement snacks"? **Rethink Your Position** *is full of bite-sized lessons on how to hold and move your body all day to nourish every one of your cells.*

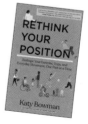